# SPIRIT OF YOUTH

## Empowering
## A New Generation

# SPIRIT OF YOUTH

## Empowering
## A New Generation

Roger Bissessar

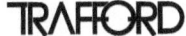

TRAFFORD

• Canada • UK • Ireland • USA •

Note for Librarians: a cataloguing record for this book that
includes Dewey Decimal Classification and US Library of
Congress numbers is available from the Library and Archives of
Canada. The complete cataloguing record can be obtained from
their online database at:
www.collectionscanada.ca/amicus/index-e.html
ISBN 1-4120-5313-7

# TRAFFORD

*Offices in Canada, USA, Ireland and UK*
This book was published *on-demand* in cooperation with
Trafford Publishing. On-demand publishing is a unique
process and service of making a book available for retail sale
to the public taking advantage of on-demand manufacturing
and Internet marketing. On-demand publishing includes
promotions, retail sales, manufacturing, order fulfilment,
accounting and collecting royalties on behalf of the author.

**Book sales for North America and international:**
Trafford Publishing, 6E–2333 Government St.,
Victoria, BC v8t 4p4 CANADA
phone 250 383 6864 (toll-free 1 888 232 4444)
fax 250 383 6804; email to orders@trafford.com
**Book sales in Europe:**
Trafford Publishing (uk) Ltd., Enterprise House,
Wistaston Road Business Centre, Wistaston Road,
Crewe, Cheshire cw2 7rp UNITED KINGDOM
phone 01270 251 396 (local rate 0845 230 9601)
facsimile 01270 254 983; orders.uk@trafford.com
**Order online at:**
trafford.com/05-0208

10 9 8 7 6 5 4 3 2

To My Dearest Shahnaaz

# ACKNOWLEDGEMENTS

I would like to express sincere thanks to my family, friends, colleagues and professional leaders for their support and encouragement towards the success of this project. The journey from 1999 November to 2004 December has indeed been a memorable one, with many challenging and exciting new experiences.

I would like to express special thanks to all my teachers in the early years at New Grant Government School and at Naparima College for laying the foundation for my literary pursuits.

To Mr. Wilton John (Director of Youth - Trinidad & Tobago), Mr. Armstrong Alexis (Regional Director - Commonwealth Youth Programme: Caribbean Centre) and Maulanaa Mustapha Kemal Hydal (Religious Head – Ahmadiyya Anjuman Isha'at I Islam Inc. of Trinidad & Tobago), thank you for the insightful discussions and your thought provoking viewpoints on so many key issues over the years.

To Mum and Dad (Mewalal & Hassina), and my brother Ryan, thank you for the wonderful memories, support and close family ties.

Sincere thanks to my wife Shahnaaz for your patience, understanding, analysis and ideas toward the successful completion of this project.

To my dear sons Raihaan & Kabir, thank you for the happiness and joy that you have brought to my life, and thanks for sharing with me your energy, vitality and fresh perspectives on the world.

Most importantly, to Almighty God, my supreme source of strength, sustenance and power, thank you for the inspiration and guidance throughout the many years of study and searching.

To all of my readers, thank you and may "Spirit of Youth – Empowering a New Generation" be a starting point in your quest for happiness, success and self-fulfillment.

# INTRODUCTION

We are all born with a higher purpose than we initially realize. As we venture through life amidst the confusion and chaos around us, this higher calling, purpose or reason dawns upon us like a flash of lighting from the heavens.

What is the true purpose of our lives? Have we ever pondered upon this question during moments of quiet and reflection? Some of us achieve significant success in terms of wealth, power and status in society but at the end of the day have we truly found peace of mind, contentment and happiness? If not, then we are like restless souls constantly driven in search of personal fulfillment, satisfaction and enlightenment.

When we reflect upon our lives, we realize that all the various personal events or situations we have experienced, whether good or bad, have shaped us into the individuals we are at this point in time. These events have shaped and moulded us into the individuals that we have become. The only constant factor in life amidst all these elements is change. We are constantly challenged by change. Further to this, more and more we are faced with tremendous uncertainty in a rapidly evolving and transforming global society.

How do we deal with these challenges? What is required for us to survive this fast paced cycle of change around us? The answer to this question lies in our discovering our true purpose or higher calling in life. No book, lecturer or philosopher can really tell us our true calling. No individual or literature can really reveal our true purpose in life. They can however provoke thought, and stimulate our conscious and subconscious minds to evaluate the situation.

After personal introspection and self analysis, this higher purpose reveals itself to us. And when this realization is achieved, we are personally motivated to pursue this calling with the best of our ability.

'Spirit of Youth – Empowering a New Generation' is a search for the higher calling in our individual lives. Its aim is to stimulate thought and to provoke introspection on our journey to self realization and personal understanding. When this goal is achieved, we can effectively deal with all negative factors, and positively uplift our lives and the lives of those around us.

# CONTENTS

## DISCOVERING THE SPIRIT

## ENHANCING THE SPIRIT

## EMPOWERING THE SPIRIT

# DISCOVERING THE SPIRIT

# 1

# IN SEARCH OF THE SPIRIT

The dawn of the third millennium signals the birth of a new era of advancement, progress and success for society. The twenty-first century represents the starting point for tremendous scientific, technological and human accomplishment and achievement. New discoveries await us. New theories will evolve. New concepts, ideas and philosophies will be the order of the day. Continuous change and transformation will face us as we strive to keep up with the pace of daily existence.

The twentieth century was indeed an amazing period of human achievement. In the realm of science and technology, we experienced an explosion of knowledge unparalleled by any other period of human existence. Mankind was able to split the atom, decode DNA, invent the computer and conquer land, air and sea with inventions such as automobiles, aeroplanes, ships and submarines. These achievements and many others serve only as an elementary stage of discovery, with further improvements, modifications and changes awaiting us in the new millennium.

With all of our accomplishments and achievements, it is interesting to note the events of 1999 and the significance of December 31, 1999 in particular. The year 1999 can be summarised as a year of anxiety, uncertainty, concern and fear. For several years before, technology experts had predicted the potential consequences of the date change over to January 01, 2000. The potential problems were referred to as the Y2K challenge. Y2K, Year 2000 Compliance, had been the buzzword of the late 1990's. Many experts had speculated on the possible consequences of Y2K, but none of them were certain.

There had been several predictions of scientific and economic chaos. The computer, one of the greatest inventions of the twentieth century was now the greatest source of fear. Almost every aspect of daily existence was linked to computers, and the effects of system non-compliance were frightening. The possibility of electrical power loss, computer system failure, loss of banking financial records and failure of nuclear systems were all perceived as a potential reality. All of these were based on the uncertainty of the date changeover.

The twentieth century had witnessed the pride of human discovery and scientific achievement. It was ironic that with all of the progress and material development of the previous one hundred years, mankind stood at the doorway of the year 2000, uncertain of the future. Our greatest scientists, philosophers, bankers, generals, teachers, politicians and leaders were unable to provide us with definite answers on the impact of Y2K and the date changeover to January 01, 2000.

So as the year 1999 progressed and December 31, 1999 finally arrived, there was tremendous uncertainty, anxiety and fear. As the night passed, and the hour drew closer, tension continued to build. We watched, waited and hoped. Within the last seconds of December 31, 1999, we held our breaths and waited to exhale. At the point of climax, when January 01, 2000 arrived, all systems were intact, and society had survived its worst fears. The lights were on, all systems were operational and we were successful in preventing global chaos. Our computer systems had conquered the test of time.

With the success of Y2K compliance, society was overflowing with joy. We held our heads up high, swelled our chests with pride and glorified our accomplishments over the past century. This was indeed a stark contrast from a couple hours before.

With the euphoria of Y2K compliance being infectious, on January 01, 2000, a global party commenced, which was unrivalled by past generations. Over one million people were celebrating in Times Square, New York. At the landmark of ancient civilisation, the Pyramids of Egypt, thousands were magnetised by a fantastic techno-laser light extravaganza. In Australia, the most spectacular fireworks display exploded in the sky over the Sydney Harbour Bridge. On the beaches of Rio de Janeiro, samba rhythms pulsated through the night as thousands partied on. On all continents of the world, people celebrated and rejoiced in every conceivable way, as mankind said goodbye to the 1900's and said hello to the new era of civilisation.

Amidst all the celebration on this glorious night, many had already forgotten the humbling experience of December 31, 1999. This period of uncertainty almost overshadowed the glorious achievements of the previous century. With all of our advancement, progress and accomplishment of the past, we had been uncertain of the future. Mankind had stood at the doorway of a new era, unable to confidently predict the events that would lie ahead. This indeed highlighted a key aspect of our existence, which was the limitation of human knowledge and our need for continuous development.

A careful study of the universe highlights perfect order, equilibrium and harmony. The laws of nature are precise, exact and fixed. Through analysis and experimentation, mankind has been able to unearth many laws of the universe, demonstrating their exactness. Philosophical minds throughout the ages have pondered on the majesty of the universe. In terms of size and space, we are almost unable to quantify it. We are in awe at the diversity of the earth we inhabit, and are humbled by the magnificence of the universe.

The eternal question in life has always been, 'What is the purpose of our existence?' Do we just exist, and at death, everything comes to and end, or is there a higher stage of life? Are we merely a physical being, or are we infinitely higher and greater? What was responsible for our creation, or more importantly, who? These questions have continuously provoked the mind of mankind, and with the arrival of the new millennium, further soul searching and introspection will continue.

One of the main lessons of the Y2K experience was that the objects created by mankind demonstrate a level of imperfection, but the laws of the universe demonstrate perfection. Is there a higher force responsible for creation and the mathematical precision of the universe?

With the dawn of the new millennium, there will be several opportunities for progress. This new era is a period of celebration, happiness and hope for a better tomorrow. We will be better poised to shape a new world order. In shaping the future, we must always remember the lessons of the past.

One of the greatest lessons of the past is to understand the purpose of our existence. We must search for wisdom and understanding of our true purpose in life and our role in society.

With all the opportunities of the twenty-first century, many of the problems of the twentieth century still remain unsolved. These problems will be carried into the new century and present a further challenge for future generations. One of our roles is to develop strategies to resolve these problems.

United Nations statistics indicate that by the year 2005, over 55% of the global population will be below the age of 30 years. The age group 12-30 years has traditionally been referred to as the youth of our society. Youth is the age of strength, beauty, energy and vitality. It is a period of transition and tremendous change, as we evolve from the stage of a child into the realm of adulthood. Our experiences, challenges and opportunities impact profoundly on our lives, and mould and shape us into the adults of tomorrow.

Different societies have different perceptions of youth. In some countries, from the time a person is 13 years old, they are considered as an adult. In other regions, the age of youth is 12-25 years, while other regions define youth as the age group 13-35 years. The United Nations defines youth as an individual within the age group 12-25 years, while the Commonwealth specification is 14-29 years.

Whatever the age specification, the question of interest is what is the Spirit of youth? Is youth limited by a mere number or is it a state of mind, a philosophical approach, or a perpetual state of existence? Our personal approach to life will determine our outlook. Some people consider themselves youthful regardless of their physical age.

Trends in society have highlighted several major issues impacting on youth. Some of these include unemployment, poverty, crime, peer pressure, sexual and reproductive health issues, lack of respect and the need for empowerment, to name a few. How do we help solve these problems? Many adults view youth as being unable to take care of themselves, lacking vision and focus and as being the cause of all these problems, but is this really so? This attitude to youth in itself is another issue to be resolved.

To attempt to deal with these problems, and many other key issues, we must first ask ourselves, do we understand our own issues? Do we fully understand our own lives and our own challenges? Who are we? Where are we going and how do we plan to get there? If we do not understand who we are, then how can we help others to truly discover themselves? If we lack direction and focus ourselves, how can we provide the direction for others?

To truly make an impact and resolve the problems of society, we must first understand ourselves. We must look within, analyse our lives, and strive to tap into our true potential and unlimited energy. We must search for inner peace and understanding of our true nature. This must be the starting point of our journey. Life is a journey, not a destination. Once we commence the journey, many exciting discoveries await us along the way. Many thrilling experiences and opportunities will lie ahead of us.

Our journey must be transformed into a search for understanding. It must be a quest to discover the purpose of our life. We were all born for a different purpose, and we need to discover our true calling. To each individual, the journey will hold different discoveries. We will discover different qualities and attributes based on our temperament and tastes. We will uncover our individual goals, dreams and aspirations. We each have a role to play, and we must work towards discovering our role and towards making a meaningful contribution to society. Only with our newly acquired knowledge can we attempt to help those around us. Only then can we attempt to resolve the problems of society. Our journey must include a search for unlocking and understanding the various aspects of the human spirit. We must strive to understand the Spirit of youth. We must commence the journey in search of the spirit.

# 2

# THE UNTAMED SPIRIT

Youth is a very magical stage of life. It is a transitional period when we move away from the innocence of childhood into the realm of becoming an adult. It is a period of inquisitiveness, transformation and exploration. We encounter new experiences that will impact profoundly upon our lives, and which lay the foundation for our future growth and progression.

Youth is characterised by an abundance of energy, vigour and vitality. During our youth, we are brimming with enthusiasm, restless and full of zest. We are very passionate, effervescent and at times uninhibited. The unbridled temperament of youth can be referred to as the Untamed Spirit. This raw, unrefined energy is one of the defining qualities of youth.

What is the general perception of youth by the adult population? The majority of adults consider youth as a problem group, lacking vision or focus, being unable to take care of themselves. The age of youth has traditionally been considered as being a period of rebellion, arrogance and resistance to those in authority. This is attributed to the restlessness so characteristic during this period of life. Most adults believe that they know what is best for youth, and attempt to dictate the pace for them to follow. This is where the conflict between the groups surfaces.

Each one of us must carefully analyse our essential nature and ask ourselves the question, "Are we youths, or are we adults? Are we youths striving to be adults, or are we adults yearning to be youths?" Many people consider youth as a state of mind, and not limited by physical age or number. Others believe that there is a clear distinction between youth and adulthood, which is clearly defined by a specific number. The answers to these questions will depend on our individual perception, attitude and experience in life, and our individual definition of both.

To provide answers in life, it is necessary to further question ourselves. What are the thoughts flowing through our minds as we face our daily experiences? Are we full of hopes and dreams, striving to make the world a better place, or are we negative and pessimistic based on our experiences and the challenges encountered? What motivates us day after day to perform our different tasks and functions in society? Are we satisfied with the lives that we lead, or do we yearn for things to be different? If we could make anything different, what would it be?

Self-analysis opens the floodgate to more questions, which provoke our minds and initiate further thought on the purpose of our existence. Whether we consider ourselves as youths or as adults will indeed be based on our experiences in life, and the level of our personal development.

At the age of youth, we are restless and easily dissatisfied by the slower pace around us. We want action and change. We crave for attention. We yearn for respect and recognition. Our boundless reservoir of energy propels us as we move though life, aiming to achieve our goals. Youth is a time for action, positive or negative. The determining factor on the type of action taken will depend on the influences acting on the life of each individual. This search for action takes us in different directions.

At the age of youth, we are curious and inquisitive, always in search of new experiences and discoveries. This curious nature can lead to either positive or negative consequences. Positive curiosity leads to a search for a greater understanding of the purpose of life. We seek to understand our individuality and our role in society. We seek to discover our full potential, and the real power of our mind. We study the problems of society and search for ways to solve them. We are curious about our past, the present and our ability to positively impact on the future. Negative curiosity can lead to a further perpetuation of the problems of society.

Trends of the twentieth century highlight many serious, unresolved problems facing the youth globally. These include alcoholism, drug abuse, unemployment, crime, sexual abuse, HIV / AIDS, poverty, illiteracy, racial discrimination and a lack of basic human rights. Many of these problems have been due to negative harnessing of the restless nature and untamed spirit of youth.

Peer pressure is one of the main factors responsible for the problems of youth. One of the basic needs of human nature is the need to belong, the need to be socially accepted. Many of us possess a strong desire to belong, and to be accepted among our peers. This need for acceptance cause many youth to experiment with new habits and to perform similar acts as the majority around them, even though it may be considered as wrong.

The identifying with popular trends in music, fashion and style in society highlights the basic need for youth to feel a sense of belonging. In the different eras of society, whether it was the 1960's, 1970's, 1980's, 1990's, fashion has been one of the defining statements of youth. Clothing, dress, hairstyles have all evolved through different cycles, each representing the voice of the youth at each period.

Different habits have been adopted by many youths, to gain popularity among friends. Drinking of alcohol, for example, even though it has been proven to have destructive effects on the body, is one of the most popular pastimes in society. A large proportion of society consumes alcohol. It is glamorised on radio, television and newspapers with sensational advertisements displaying popularity and fame. This indeed is promoted as socially acceptable.

Drinking of alcohol among youth is condemned, but is practised by the adults in society. Does a double standard not arise in the minds of youth when adults tell them not to drink? Indeed it would seem so. Many of us around the globe consume alcohol. It is considered as glamorous, sophisticated and ultra-cool. To face the threat of being unpopular, being laughed at or ridiculed for not wanting to partake in the festivities, how many of us will take a stand and not follow the crowd? The peer pressure is usually too great, and many are unable to take a stand against drinking, and eventually give in.

Youth and sexuality is another area where many find themselves in very compromising situations. At the early stages of youth, we are now discovering our sexuality. Our sexual energy begins to blossom and hormonal changes cause a flood of emotional and sexual changes. Our inability to understand and control this new energy can cause devastating consequences. One of the main problems of the last century was the spread of AIDS due to the HIV virus. Promiscuity, lack of sexual restraint, unprotected sex were some of the factors contributing to this critical problem. The challenge of the new millennium will not only entail discovering a cure for HIV / AIDS, but creating a greater level of sexual awareness and maturity in society.

Crime is another area of tremendous concern within the last century. The frightening aspects of the statistics highlight that the major crimes are being performed by youth within the age group 13 – 29. Why have so many youth turned to crime? Is it because we have failed as a society to provide proper avenues for moral and social development? Have the problems of unemployment and poverty forced youth to take alternative action to provide for their families and their loved ones? Are the youth that are involved in crime inherently bad, or is it that circumstances in life have not provided avenues for their development? We must carefully seek to determine the cause of these trends, as we aim to provide answers to these issues.

For the youth in search of friends, in search of belonging, the habits of the majority become acceptable. If everyone is drinking alcohol, smoking cigarettes or marijuana and indulging in promiscuous behaviour, then this appears glamorous and becomes attractive and acceptable to the individual. This lays the foundation for a matrix of problems to develop. This complicated web of social issues will generate many challenges for society to resolve.

What is the cause of so many youth giving in to the peer pressure around them? The root cause is a lack of self-confidence and low self-esteem. Individuals who are confident, self-assured and assertive will never compromise their personal values because of peer pressure. At the risk of being unpopular, these individuals will prefer to stand alone in their beliefs, rather than give in to the practices of the masses. How can we curb the impact of peer pressure on youths? The starting point on this road to recovery will entail building the self-confidence and self- esteem of youth and helping them to feel good about themselves and who they are. Each one of us is special and unique in our own way. We have a right to express our ideas and beliefs, and should never be intimidated by those around us. We must confidently assert our presence in society, fearless of the taunting of others.

Youth must be made to realise their tremendous value, worth and infinite potential for positive advancement and progress. They must be made aware of their ability to create a better life for themselves and their loved ones through positive habits and practices. This will serve as the first stage on the path of progress. Avenues need to be developed to allow youth to positively express themselves. Proper Counselling services, Peer Guidance and Volunteer programs should be established to help youths who require advice and guidance on dealing with personal problems.

The second step will involve enhancement of the communication and inter-relationship between youth and adults. Traditionally, adults have viewed youth as unable to plan for themselves, and as always requiring direction and guidance. A significant change in attitude is required among the adult population of the new millennium. Youth must be recognised for their potential for progress, and must be empowered to become masters of their own destiny. Proper training and guidance is required for the adults, to help them to change their outlook towards youth.

Youth are overflowing with energy, vitality and passion. This creative energy must be positively harnessed to achieve the desired goals. At the stage of youth, the untamed spirit manifests itself as raw, unrefined energy. If this energy is left unchecked, destructive consequences can occur. If the energy is overly controlled, individual growth will be inhibited and rebellion will occur. An optimum balance of nurturing the spirit, with a sense of self-respect is required to achieve true development. Through the process of positively harnessing the potential of the untamed spirit, tremendous benefits will be achieved for our youth. We must all work towards taking the process from mere academic theory to a practical reality.

# 3

# THE ATHLETIC SPIRIT

The arena of sports provides valuable opportunities for expression of the human spirit. Whether it is in football, cricket, basketball, track and field, swimming, cycling or gymnastics, we learn some of the most valuable lessons in life through sports. Some of the most magical moments in history have manifested themselves through sports. Alive in the minds of many are the golden images of athletic success, captured in a single moment that transcends the barrier of time, living on for eternity.

Sport has the potential to be one of the greatest unifying forces of mankind. It has the unique ability to make people forget national and international conflicts, and creates opportunities for togetherness, harmony and brotherhood. Whether we are athletes or spectators, sports can have a tremendous impact on our lives. We forget personal, family and national problems, and focus on bringing out the best qualities and are able to enjoy the events as they unfold.

We all possess an athletic spirit. The level of expression of this spirit varies with each individual in society. It is dormant in some people, but highly developed in others. Innate in all of us is the potential to exert ourselves to the best of our ability. Latent within us is the desire to physically express ourselves, and to partake in sports either for pleasure, relaxation, exercise or serious competition. The athletic spirit not only manifests itself on the playing field, but also transcends into our daily lives. It is present in our attitude to life and our aiming to be the best at what we endeavour.

We learn many vital lessons from the realm of sports. We feel the thrill of victory, the exhilaration and excitement of being a winner, and being recognised as the best. We experience the thrill of conquering the event, defeating our fellow competitors. We realize the rewards of discipline, proper planning, training, focus and direction.

Another lesson we learn is the agony of defeat. Sometimes we taste defeat after battling with our fellow competitors. We may have given of our best personal performance, but it was not enough to be declared the winner. Whether we represent a town, city or country, the experience of defeat is a humbling one. This can place a heavy burden on our shoulders, as we feel that we have disappointed everyone who believed in us and who invested their time, energy and effort. We have to learn from the experience and work towards improving ourselves.

Victory and defeat provide different opportunities for our personal development and growth. The experience of victory must not boost our egos to the point where we look down upon others, becoming arrogant and obnoxious. Victory must be expressed with sportsman like behaviour and with a spirit of thanksgiving for having accomplished success. On the other side, defeat must not be looked upon as the end of the road for us. Defeat represents a starting point for improvement, and is fertile ground for sowing the seeds of future success.

In any sport there are winners and losers. In the true sense of the event, everyone who took part can be considered a winner. Participation is an important component of all events. There is however only room for one overall winner, the one that has achieved the best performance. By our very nature, defeat is not an easy experience to deal with. We feel dejected, depressed and disoriented when we do not achieve our goals. We blame ourselves, and criticise our mistakes and the mistakes of others as contributing to our failure. This is an unhealthy approach to our personal disappointments.

As highlighted before, defeat provides fertile ground for achieving future improvement and success. A careful analysis of the root cause of our failure will provide us with valuable guidance on the path to improvement. It is necessary for us all to experience defeat at some point of our lives, to provide us with opportunities for self-analysis and introspection. We must not view defeat in a negative light, but from a positive perspective. This will ensure that we experience a process of rebuilding and achieve positive growth and change.

Another lesson that we learn from sports is the value of teamwork. In all team sports, we must work together to achieve a synergistic blend of our collective talents. Individual needs are sacrificed; the main focus is what is best for the common good of the team. It is only through co-operation, sharing and unselfishness can we contribute to the goals and requirements of the team. This attitude must be carried with us off the playing field and into our daily lives. We must become team players in our endeavours.

In the realm of sports, we learn the value of hard work,

discipline, focus, determination and drive. We learn to set goals and to develop strategic plans to achieve our targets. We learn to continuously improve our performance and to become more confident and assured of our abilities. We are better able to translate these lessons in our daily lives. What are some of the ways that sports teaches us important lessons in life? One example is in the sport of football where strategic thinking and planning is critical. The defensive players of the team will pass the ball to their midfielders. The ball is gradually worked pass the opposition and then passed to the forward strikers. Through skill and talent the defence of the opposition is out-manoeuvred and the striker kicks the ball at goal, which beats the goalkeeper and scores.

This build up from defence to attack involves careful strategy and planning. Each team will study the other teams style, structure and formation. A review of their individual strengths and weaknesses will be performed. Videos of their previous matches highlighting their game plan and performance will be studied. The foundation for winning a game can be laid before the teams meet on the playing field. By knowing the opponent's strengths and weaknesses, and understanding your team and yourself, the chance of success is significantly improved. In life itself, this strategic approach must become a practical way of existence as we build our ideas from stage unto stage until they become a reality.

Through sports we learn the value of healthy lifestyles. A successful athlete must nourish the physical body to achieve optimum performance at all times. Further to this, the athlete must be nourished mentally with proper thinking and attitude. The rigours of training, continuous practice and preparation for sporting events require a high level of endurance and stamina. Physical fitness combined with healthy mental habits and thought processes are essential for all round development of the individual.

The importance of training is highlighted in all avenues of sport. It is only through dedication and continuous practice that we perfect the skills and talents required for athletic success. Through the vital lessons that we learn in sports, the raw energy of the untamed spirit can be transformed into positive energy via the athletic spirit. This is a manifestation of the focused energy of the total human spirit.

One of the most spectacular and exhilarating displays of the power of sports is witnessed every four years via the Olympic Games. From Athens Greece in 1896, through different global venues to Athens again in 2004, the Olympic Games have highlighted the infinite potential of the human spirit. During these games opportunities have been provided for some of the poorest countries, and least known individuals to rise to fame and glory through superior athletic performance. In the realm of track and field, gymnastics, swimming, team events, heroes and heroines have emerged who have left breathtaking moments locked within our minds for eternity. This glory will once again be achieved in China 2008 and in future Olympic games.

Many athletes have been able to achieve personal success and glory for their country over the years. Some of these individuals include Carl Lewis, Nadia Comaneci, Jackie Joyner Kersee and Ian Thorpe, as just a few of the many legends who have written their names into Olympic history.

In the realm of the Olympic Games, opportunities have been provided for significant political statements and views to be expressed. Once such moment occurred at the Sydney Olympics 2000 when Cathy Freeman won the 400 m gold medal. This signalled a victory not only for her, but a victory for the struggle of the Aboriginal people of Australia throughout the ages. When Jesse Owens won the 100 m gold medal at the Berlin Olympics in 1936 during Nazi reign, this sent a powerful racial statement throughout the world about the equality of the human race. Many individual performances throughout the decades have been able to champion the cause of different generations.

The opportunity to represent your country at an international event is a great honour for any athlete. The glory is even greater when the individual performs well and success is achieved. In the Olympic realm, the athletic spirit rises to new heights and climaxes with the realisation of personal dreams.

Another majestic display of the athletic spirit occurs every four years in the realm of World Cup football. From the dawn of this competition in Uruguay 1930, to the most recent World Cup in Japan / Korea 2002, the world has been thrilled by the stunning display of skill, energy, talent and determination. From the Samba style of Brazil, to the precision and efficiency of Germany, the battles on the football field have exhilarated us for ages. Can we remember some of these magical moments which created heroes like Pele, Beckenbauer, Rossi, Maradonna, Romario, Mattheus, Zidane and Owen to name a few? These and many others have all become immortal by their World Cup football accomplishments and glory.

The battles of World Cup football can cause euphoria to sweep across a county, or plunge a nation into mourning. The passion, energy and spirit of this event transcend the limits of other global events. The final outcomes of matches have a powerful and potent impact on the people of the respective countries. In South America for example, football is revered like religion. The results of World Cup Football can lead to national pride, joy and happiness or tremendous sadness and depression. The electricity and excitement of World Cup Football is phenomenal, transforming the world into a frenzy of emotions every four years.

Individual and team success in sports is of tremendous benefit to society. Sporting heroes and heroines cause joy to be spread throughout the country. People are able to forget their problems for a while. They are able to believe in themselves again, have new hopes and dreams about their ability to conquer the future. Society achieves a positive lift, as people are able to gain a positive outlook on life. For the individual athlete, the reward of hard work, dedication and commitment is personal achievement and glory. Based on their personal history, this will have special meaning to their lives. When our athletes succeed, the entire nation celebrates.

From the lessons of history, we realise the significant benefit of sports for the development of society. Sports must be used as a tool to promote physical, mental and spiritual well-being of our youth. The positive influence of the lessons of sports will contribute meaningfully towards individual development. Through sports, the vitality and energy of youth will have a healthy medium for positive expression. Sports must be promoted as a means of developing our youth and helping us to harness the positive energy that is latent within all of us.

Countries should work towards developing proper infrastructure and programs for development of youth via sports. Focus must be placed on poor youth, in rural districts, that face limited access to facilities for personal development. Proper programs and facilities will nurture the talent of our youth. Governments and the private corporate sector should recognise the value of investing in systems that will harness the most valuable resource of the nation, which is our human potential.

In the realm of sports, there never really are any losers. Once we have exerted ourselves to the best of our ability, we can all consider ourselves as winners. We transcend into a higher realm of existence when we derive the true benefits of sports. We achieve greater maturity, understanding and personal growth when we learn important lessons from sports. We achieve a natural high as we move into the higher stage of development.

Motivation of our youth to embrace the opportunities created by sports must be encouraged. Within this realm lies a valuable tool for the positive development of youth. This will allow us to create a positive impact on society in the years to come. Personal development will allow youth to implement change for the improvement of their lives, and the lives of those around us. Optimum development of the Athletic Spirit will stir us into realising our infinite potential for advancement, progress and success.

# 4

# THE COMPETITIVE SPIRIT

One of the essential aspects of human nature is our desire to be the very best at what we do. In all of our endeavours, we strive for superiority, wanting to be recognised as number one. Whether it is in sports, business, entertainment, religion, education, politics or many other aspects of our daily existence, people are always aiming to be the best. This attitude highlights the attribute of our existence known as the Competitive Spirit.

The Competitive Spirit can impact upon us either negatively or positively. The negative aspects highlight themselves when we are willing to employ immoral or unlawful methods to accomplish our goals. Depending on our yearning for success, we may resort to any means necessary for the desired result. The positive aspect of the spirit is based on our working to positively develop ourselves physically, mentally and spiritually as we strive to be the best at what we do. Our efforts must be directed to constructive change in the world around us

From a very early stage of life, we are engulfed in a competitive outlook towards our daily affairs. From our early days at school, we compete for top marks in the classroom, yearning to be recognized as the smartest and best student. As we progress through different stages of our education, competition becomes more intense in our pursuit of academic progress. Our acceptance into schools, colleges or universities all depend on our overall performance.

When we graduate from secondary or tertiary education, we compete with other people for interviews to gain employment. When we gain employment, we strive to stay ahead of everyone else. We work very hard to gain promotions, salary increases, improved benefits and opportunities. As we progress professionally, we need to continually improve our skills and overall marketability. It is essential for us to be on a path of continuous learning, always furthering our education, pursuing post- graduate studies, attending training seminars and refresher courses. We always need to be in a mode of capacity building and continuous development.

If we become entrepreneurs, it is even more critical for us to continually improve our performance and demonstrate excellence. In a shrinking market for professional services, with rapid advances and changes in technology, we must offer more value for customer investment and stay ahead of our competitors. To be successful, we must be constantly competing with other companies for the limited contracts available, and provide optimum benefits to our clients.

In the realm of entertainment, competition for the paying audience is intense. Whether it is in the film, television, music or theatre industry, entertainers continually need to captivate their audience with their best performances. Entertainment companies are constantly searching for new concepts, ideas and innovations to capture the interest of the audience. Significant investment is focused on this industry to harness state-of-the-art techniques, special effects and technology to ensure audience satisfaction. The end result of this investment includes high quality entertainment, customer satisfaction and maximum capital return for the investor. Another aspect of this industry can even include competition for official awards recognizing the best entertainment production.

In the field of politics, there is significant competition for the support of the people and for votes on Election Day. Politicians and political parties compete for the support of the population. They attempt to satisfy the needs of the population, within the limits of existing programmes, policies and available funding. At the end of the day, the most popular politician and political party is the one perceived by the people to best represent and fulfil their needs. The politician best able to obtain the majority of support will officially represent the people in political office.

Even in the sphere of religion, we witness competition between various philosophies. Each religious group declares itself as possessing the best philosophical ideology, the best religious scripture, the best spiritual leader. There is competition between groups to convert people to different faiths and to different belief systems. This competition stirs emotional responses and can foster hatred, instead of promoting peace and goodwill. Sometimes even within the same religious faith, there is competition between groups, because of different interpretations of certain aspects of the religion.

Competition for land is another issue we witness in our daily lives. Whether it is in a village, town, city, country or inter-country, the dispute for land can lead to severe consequences. Significant wars, sanctions, conflicts and battles have occurred internationally due to the fight and claim for land by different groups. History highlights this as a prevalent trend among countries.

Competition is indeed the name of the game. Some of us revel in this way of life, enjoying the excitement. Others may fall by the wayside, unable to keep up with the fast pace of living. By our very nature, we are competitive beings. We need to satisfy our egos. We need to accomplish success in our endeavours. We need to be recognised as the very best. This attitude and outlook on life are characteristic of a Competitive Spirit.

The pressure of competition can cause individuals to resort to alternative means to achieve success. People are sometimes unable to cope with the thought of being second best. This is the reason why some athletes may take steroids or performance-enhancing drugs. They need to win at all costs. This desire outweighs the consequences of being caught, or the ill-effects on their bodies.

This is the reason why some students may copy during an examination, or buy examination papers beforehand. The need to pass an examination can outweigh the consequences of being expelled. In an effort to generate additional income and achieve quick financial success, businesses often feel the pressure of competition. To overcome this pressure, some may engage in illegal practices, for instance, bribing politicians in order to receive political favours or not adhering to proper accounting practises.

Further negative aspects are highlighted by gang violence among youths, in an effort to claim supremacy. Each gang wants to be the strongest, the most feared, the very best. One of the reasons for drug violence and wars between drug cartels is competition for control of a particular territory. Fierce competition between such groups have devastating consequences on some countries including kidnapping, murder and acts of terrorism.

Competition can be healthy or disastrous. The net effect is determined by the circumstances, the issues and the individuals involved. Our ability to manage competition is essential in our level of progress and personal development, and by extension, our impact on society. The Competitive Spirit is an integral aspect of youth, and in order to gain further insight into our true nature, we must first understand the power of the spirit.

Of all the different aspects of competition that exist, there is one critical area that we continue to neglect - competition against ourselves. Many of us focus on competing against each other, but do not realise that we need to focus on competing against ourselves.

Competition against our self is one of the most potent avenues of self-development and progress. We must continually strive for physical, mental and spiritual elevation and progress. We must always seek to improve our physical health, increase our knowledge, and achieve greater understanding of the world we live in. We must work towards achieving inner peace, self-fulfilment and wisdom. It is only when we have achieved understanding of our purpose in life, can we help others to find happiness and meaning out of life. Only then can we fully work towards improving our own conditions and the conditions of society.

We must constantly assess our stage of existence and personal development, at different periods of our lives. Using this as a starting point, we can set new standards, goals and milestones. By adopting an approach of self-development, competition can be used positively for our personal development and for the development of those around us.

We need to perform a gap analysis highlighting our personal weaknesses and deficiencies. First of all, we need to determine our personal knowledge base, skills and educational qualifications. Using this information as a reference, we can work towards acquisition of new knowledge and skills, and embark on a path of further personal, academic and professional development. The positive technique of competing against ourselves will continually contribute towards our progress and improvement. By our nature we thrive on competition, and positive competition propels us to higher achievements.

After a particular point in time, based on an accumulation of our experiences and personal development, our maximum performance will be limited by our level of development. This performance can be improved by altering our training or embarking on new techniques and strategies. This continuous process of assessment and evaluation is a critical tool on the path to self-advancement.

In the realm of sports, athletes must first establish their best personal performance, based on their present level of development. With this information, a proper training programme and schedule can be developed to ensure that improved personal performance and fitness are achieved. With further development, and as we improve, new milestones and targets will continually be achieved.

Using the psychology of competition, we will achieve positive development of the human spirit. We will significantly reduce the time taken for our daily tasks, improve physical fitness and initiate further mental development and spiritual well being. We will increase our knowledge and improve our personal and professional skills. Through proper harnessing of the competitive spirit, we will positively impact on our environment, and be of significant benefit to our global community.

# 5

# THE ARTISTIC SPIRIT

Through the medium of paint, cloth, wood, stone, bronze, silver or gold, art is a means of expression of the human soul. Using the realm of painting, sculpture, carving, poetry or music, artists have been able to reveal their inner most thoughts, feelings and secrets. Throughout history, some of the greatest artistic masterpieces were due to the creative and expressive energy of our talented artists.

The fine works of art throughout the ages are a manifestation of our latent creativity and artistic spirit. As we venture into the realm of youth, we realise that there is a tremendous creative energy waiting to be expressed through the medium of art. Throughout the ages, art has evolved and been able to capture the mood, feelings and events of society at each point of our history and development. The evolution of society is captured by the artists of each generation.

Art is a manifestation of human skill, initiative and imagination design as witnessed in painting, architecture, language, music and other fields of human endeavour. Every one of us possesses artistic qualities and ability. What varies is the level of development of these skills, and our belief in our ability to express them. Some people demonstrate natural talent and ability, while others require training to realise their hidden abilities.

The youth of society possess tremendous energy and vitality that drives them in their daily activities. Without proper avenues for expression, this energy can cause them to feel restless and unfulfilled. Art is a valuable mechanism for expression of the energy of youth. Through art, our youth will be able to express their thoughts, moods and feelings. This opportunity for expression will allow the views, feelings and emotions of youth to be heard.

Through art, our youth can make a statement on the state of affairs in their community or country. The problem of environmental destruction, for example, can be captured in painting, where the artist highlights scenes reflecting our destruction of the earth. The powerful message of visual expression serves as an effective means of sensitising people to problems facing society, and the need for change in our habits, lifestyles and relations with each other.

What motivates us to create art? What are the lessons we derive from the work of an artist? Art is a means of our expression and imitation of real life. The painting or sculpture, for example, is merely an imitation of real objects that are being portrayed. Through the different art forms, artists are able to express their reverence for nature or respect for great human personalities. Artists are able to express their feelings towards key issues and present their personal philosophies on life. A channel is provided to communicate their feelings to society.

Art provides testimony of the higher qualities of the human being, compared to the animal world. Indeed, we witness breath-taking works of art in the animal world, such as the manufacture of honey by the bees or the weaving of a web by a spider. These, however, are the products of instinct demonstrated by these animals, driven by fixed laws of nature. The human being, however, through the power of choice, consciously decides to create art. We consciously decide whether we are going to create or destroy.

In our lowest state of existence, we resemble the animals, acting on instinct. By demonstrating the power of choice, the power to create and use art to express our ideas, thoughts and feelings, we demonstrate our superiority over the animal world.

Painting has been one of the most popular forms of expression by artists throughout the ages. From the earliest drawings found in the caves of ancient civilisation, through the artistic explosion of the Renaissance, up to the present day abstract art, painting has demonstrated the tremendous artistic capacity of the human spirit. The works of Leonardo da Vinci, Rembrandt, Pablo Picasso and other luminaries are testimony of the pure genius and skill of the human spirit.

Sculptures are another demonstration of human endeavour, talent and skill. Sculptors have been successful in mirroring the world before them. These works highlight precision, symmetry and skill in portraying the real objects of life. Sculpting also demonstrates the ability to convert basic raw material into a product of higher worth, value and artistic beauty. An ordinary piece of wood, rock, marble, stone or bronze can be transferred into a spectacular imitation of the real world that we live in.

The works of many great artists adorn the museums and

art galleries of the world. These are a source of adoration and admiration by society. Behind each painting, drawing or sculpture, there is a particular message or meaning that the artist wishes to convey. This is their means of sharing their thoughts and ideas for the benefit of society. These masterpieces also capture the mood, feeling and thinking of artists at various points in time, helping us to better understand previous generations.

Artists who are skilful with words have produced some of the greatest pieces of literature, poetry and plays throughout the ages. One of the most famous of these was William Shakespeare, who has left us with a legacy of comedy, tragedy, drama and philosophy enveloped within his plays. These dramatic works capture a diverse range of philosophy and introspection, including our search for personal understanding and overcoming personal challenges and difficulties.

The written word is one of the most potent and powerful forms of expressing and conveying ideas. Through the written word, authors have been able to express their personal philosophy, ideology and analysis of life. Different authors attempt to stir us into contemplation and reflection upon the real purpose of our existence. Whatever the subject or the issue, authors have skilfully used words to convey their ideas to society.

In the realm of theatre, playwrights have been able to deal with controversial subjects in society. An example of this can be seen with gay issues, homosexual and lesbian lifestyles. Due to fear of condemnation from society, people with these lifestyles may be unable to openly express themselves about their sexual preferences and attitudes. In the form of a play, however, these issues can be dealt with. Society becomes more educated and better prepared to examine these issues via the literary realm.

The playwright can create characters in a play that explore the theme of gay lifestyles and the concerns involved. The attitude of parents, employers and society can be dealt with. Normally, members of the audience will not objectively review these subjects because of the setting. However, in the form of the play, they are receptive to the dialogue presented by the actors and gain new understanding and awareness. This technique is effective in sensitising society to important and relevant issues impacting on our daily lives.

Television programmes and movies present strong visual images which impact upon us subliminally. The power of audio-visual technology and special effects creates a lasting impact on our mental dynamics. Our exposure to drama, adventure, comedy, science fiction and thrillers stimulate our thoughts, emotions and feelings.

One of the most powerful forms of communication in the world today is the power of music. Music is the universal language, which transcends all barriers of language, colour, class or race. The harmony, rhythm and vibrations expressed by the musician stir our emotions and moods. The energy, passion and fire of musicians are captured in pop, rock, alternative, latin, jazz, classical, reggae, calypso, soul and other forms of music from around the world.

Music can bring us joy or sadness. We can laugh or we can cry. The rhythmic sounds can cause us to dance, and forget all the troubles in the world. The harmonious sounds of musicians reverberate in our minds. The powerful lyrics of the composers create a profound impact on society at different periods of time and can significantly influence our youths.

There are songs that have stirred violence, sexual misconduct, and even suicide. The messages from the lyrics can be potent. We need to utilise music to positively impact on our youth. Our artistes need to express positive messages, to create positive changes in attitudes, lifestyles and behaviour in society. If there is anyone that youth will listen to, it is their favourite musicians. A well co-ordinated programme with global artistes and musicians will create positive change for society.

With the rapid advancement of technology over the last decade, there are new and innovative avenues for artistic expression. In the virtual realm, through computer programmes and software, graphic artists are creating artwork through this new medium. With the advent of internet technology and the World Wide Web, web sites are created daily with different visual impact and layout to appeal to the global population. The webmasters are artists behind the scenes.

The youth of society possess tremendous artistic talent waiting to be unleashed. History bears testimony to the legacy of young artists. The energy and fire of youth can be channelled into realm of art and artistic expression. Many youths already display natural talent, others require further training. Proper guidance and support must be provided for young, budding artists. Mechanisms must be in place to allow for their nurturing and development. This will impact positively on our youth, allowing for optimum mental, emotional and spiritual development. We will be able to realise our higher capabilities and talent by unleashing the artistic spirit.

Art can positively contribute towards enhancing the self-confidence of youth. After working very hard to create a particular art form, the young artist gains personal satisfaction from creating a finished product from an initial idea. A new sense of self-esteem and worth is gained from developing a creation that impacts on society. This gain in self-confidence and self-worth will lead to a more positive attitude and life-style for the individual, and allow them to strive for further improvement and growth in their lives. In contemplating the power of art, we must always understand the tremendous impact of music upon youth. Of all the factors of society, music is one of the most powerful forces acting upon youth. Youths identify with particular songs, musicians and messages that capture their mood. We idolise and revere our favourite artistes. We copy their hairstyles, behaviour, fashion and habits. We are influenced, directly or subliminally, by our favourite performers.

Each generation has it's own musical icon. From the era of Elvis, the Beatles and Frank Sinatra, through the period of Prince, Michael Jackson, Madonna and George Michael, to the present reverence for Shakira, Britney Spears, Jennifer Lopez, Puff Daddy, Eminem and Beyonce, there will always be artistes who are idolised by the masses. Their music, image and aura have transformed behaviour, fashion, style and attitudes in society. This power will always belong to the musician. Up to this very day, the music of many deceased musicians still echo in our hearts, mind and soul. From the rebel cry of Bob Marley, to the reflection of John Lennon, to the raw passion of Elvis Presley, we experience the personality of our favourite artistes forever in their music. We must never underestimate the power of music.

Art is a valuable means of expressing creativity and innovation for the benefit of society. As we journey through life in search of greater understanding, we must strive to unlock the artistic spirit within all of us. In this way, we will discover new dimensions and realms, and gain greater insight into our true nature and the higher purpose of our existence.

Art is more than a manifestation of the mind. It is an expression of the human spirit. The early stages of youth deal with our physical development. The later stages allow for our mental, emotional and spiritual development. Art can positively contribute towards our holistic evolution, development and maturity. Searching to discover our artistic spirit will empower us to take control of our lives, and become more assertive and self-confident. It will elevate our self-esteem and allow us to impact positively on the lives of those around us.

# 6

# THE ENTREPRENEURIAL SPIRIT

With the rapid advancement of technology, restructuring and re-engineering of organisations, corporate mergers, retrenchment, voluntary separation and early retirement, unemployment has reached significant levels globally. With these continuous trends, unemployment is one of the main challenges facing the world today. How can society adapt to these changes and what measures are required to resolve this situation? The answer to this question lies in understanding the true essence of the human spirit.

The human spirit possesses the ability to shape the future, to control our destiny, to create a new reality from nothing. Based on where we are in life, we can determine where would like to be and how we plan to get there. In times of economic change and chaos, organizational transformation, corporate restructuring and tough employment challenges, we need to unlock the dimension within us known as the Entrepreneurial Spirit.

What is an entrepreneur? What are the qualities that such an individual must possess? An entrepreneur is one who possesses the ability to create employment for themselves and for others. The entrepreneurial spirit is characterized by vision, initiative, persistence and personal drive. Defining qualities of such an individual include commitment to work, creativity, being goal-oriented and willingness to take risks. We all possess the entrepreneurial spirit, the secret is to discover our true calling.

Many of us possess very good ideas, but are fearful of the future and the risks involved in implementing them. We lack the self-confidence required to promote our ideas and lack the decision making skills required to take calculated business risks. We are comfortable with our existing jobs and employment opportunities, but secretly dream about owning our own business. Within our minds are good ideas and concepts for new business opportunities, but we are unwilling to take the first step on the path to making these thoughts a reality.

What are some of the questions we must ask to determine our entrepreneurial ability? Do we possess the determination to finish what we have started? Can we work well with others? Are we good at organizing, communicating and motivating others? Are we imaginative, creative and good at problem solving? Are we innovative? Is our thinking holistic? Are we calm under pressure? If we answered yes to all of these questions, the entrepreneurial spirit is alive and well. If not, re-awakening of the spirit is required through motivation to increase self-confidence.

We must reflect and ask ourselves, what are the qualities of a good entrepreneur? The individual must possess determination, drive, energy and persistence. The individual needs to be decisive, action oriented, solution oriented, systematic and willing to take calculated risks. Very strong skills in strategic planning and long term forecasting will also be critical skills.

A good entrepreneur harnesses creativity, imagination and vision to offer original ideas and concepts to society. Demonstrated must be a high level of self-confidence, convincing marketing skills, and the ability to positively motivate others. A high level of flexibility and the ability to learn valuable lessons from mistakes will be other key assets. An ability to adapt to change and a willingness to explore new techniques, concepts and strategies are key characteristics of a good entrepreneur.

One of the critical ingredients for entrepreneurial success is sound technical knowledge in the field of activity. Possession of strong technical knowledge in the chosen field, demonstrated competence and the ability to perform the required tasks make the difference between success or failure. It is essential for the entrepreneur to be innovative, proactive and up-to-date with the latest advances in technology, products and services in the chosen field.

Based on the level of technological advancement and progress of society, many people believe that there are not many new ideas left to be discovered. Nothing could be further from the truth. As we move through the new millennium, we must always realize that there are new concepts, ideas and discoveries waiting to be unveiled. As society advances, there will be continuous change, continuous discovery and the evolution of new strategies for continuous improvement.

The entrepreneur of the twenty-first century must embrace the new tools available for business success. In a global village, with internet technology, web sites, e-commerce, there are tremendous opportunities for marketing our products, skills and services. Computers and cyber technology provide the vital link for communication, information transfer and customer contact.

The biggest obstacle to entrepreneurial success is fear. The fear of failure, fear of making mistakes, fear of venturing into the unknown are critical obstacles to our progress. Fear cripples and inhibits us from truly expressing ourselves. We need to eliminate fear and replace it with faith, hope and belief. We need to demonstrate confidence in our ability to achieve success, and to make our dreams a reality.

Belief in our ability is the catalyst towards implementing positive change and to unleashing the entrepreneurial spirit. There is an ancient Chinese proverb that states, "Give a man a fish, feed him for a day. Teach a man to fish, feed him for life." Empowering people to learn a new skill and to increase their self-confidence and sense of self-worth will guide them unto the path of self-sustenance and positive change.

Entrepreneurial nurturing and development is a valuable mechanism for empowering youth in the new millennium. The symbol of entrepreneurship is confident, empowered youth, who strongly believe in their ability to positively mould, shape and influence the future. The creation of new business ventures based on entrepreneurial ideas will be a source of creating employment. New business generates employment and motivates others to pursue their own ideas and dreams.

Youth in society possess an abundance of talent and skills waiting to be tapped. Many have achieved significant academic success, while others demonstrate tremendous skill in the field of art, craft and vocational subjects. Several of these individuals end up working for different companies which are struggling for economic survival and continuously cutting cost via retrenchment and downsizing. With the harsh market conditions, many youths are generally the first to be laid off during these periods of downsizing caused by global mergers, re-engineering and change in organizational philosophy. This contributes significantly to high unemployment rates.

Youth need to be provided with avenues for entrepreneurial training and guidance to develop and market their individual skills and services. More institutions and programs must be established to provide entrepreneurial guidance and assistance to youth. This would include financial training, start-up funding and mentoring programs. Government policy must cater specifically for nurturing young entrepreneurs. Special incentives, interest rates, repayment rates must be made available for these young entrepreneurs to seed and grow new business ventures.

The establishment of programs and incentives specifically for youth will provide significant benefit to society. Improvement in the economy, reduction in unemployment and increase in self-confidence of the new generation of entrepreneurs are a few of the rewards to be achieved. The level of success of these businesses will create further indirect employment and spin off industries.

The innovative ideas, services and new concepts expressed through youth entrepreneurial activity will stimulate further economic activity and progress. The creation of new employment will incrementally reduce crime and provide for positive social change. Harnessing the entrepreneurial spirit will provide significant opportunities for the advancement and progress of society. The way forward will be to provide meaningful opportunities for young entrepreneurs to prosper.

# 7

# THE POSITIVE SPIRIT

Many people in the world today are depressed, disoriented and dissatisfied with life. They are discontented with their jobs, their level of education, their health, wealth, personal achievements and other aspects of their daily existence. They are very miserable and unhappy. Daily existence for them is a struggle. What is the root cause of this severe depression and general unhappiness? The answer to this question lies in our state of mind and attitude and outlook towards life.

In our daily lives, each one of us faces many diverse challenges. We are faced with different trials and tribulations. What is our attitude to these situations and how do we deal with these different issues? Our mental outlook and attitude towards these challenges will determine our level of success in overcoming them.

Many of us possess a negative outlook in life, and to the situations that we face. We create a negative state of mind that limits our progress and advancement. We all possess the potential to conquer all challenges and to deal constructively with obstacles in our path. Realization of our true potential will unleash the Positive Spirit that lies dormant within us.

When we review the physical and mental realm, we realize that action is a product of thought. Our actions are physical manifestations of the thoughts that our minds dwell upon. Our ability or inability to take action is directly related to our thought processes and personal belief systems. Careful analysis of the actions of different people provides insight into their thoughts and mental dynamics. A high percentage of society possesses low self-confidence and low self-esteem. They are unable to see success as their birthright, but instead view success in life as restricted and reserved for others. This attitude manifests itself as a low sense of self-worth and inability to take action to achieve goals. This is the cause of limited success for many people in society.

Our thought patterns create our personality and the type of individuals that we become. Constant repeated thought becomes engraved in our minds and manifests themselves into the habits we develop. Just as a physical river erodes and cuts channels into the land, so too does repeated thought cut channels into our minds causing us to follow fixed paths of thinking.

Through the power of thought, we possess the ability to shape our destiny. Thought is a creative force which shapes, moulds and directly influences the future. It is a manifestation of our mental vibrations, which surge forth from the inner recesses of our mind. Our mental vibrations penetrate into the physical realm, becoming a reality and building the world around us. The mind is magnetic in nature. Whether our thoughts are positive or negative, we will experience what our minds dwell upon. Negative thoughts attract negative expectations and that which we fear. Positive thoughts attract our positive expectations and that which we desire. We must learn to focus the mind positively, to attract positive desires and to create positive experiences.

If we constantly live in fear, we attract that which we fear. If we learn to practice faith, we can develop the art of attracting that which we have faith in. To realize the full power of the mind and the vitality of the positive spirit, we must first understand the potency of our thought patterns. Many people understand the impact of food on the physical body and can easily go on a physical diet. Few understand the influence of thought on the mental realm, and the need to go on a mental diet. The mental realm is influenced by our mental input and output. We need to control our thoughts and be careful what we allow our minds to continuously dwell upon. Implementing a mental diet will allow us to achieve positive goals and desires.

One of the major factors impacting upon our thought is our external environment. The people we associate with, the newspapers we read, the radio programs we listen to, the television programs that we view, all impact upon us subliminally. The powerful messages from these diverse audio-visual media impact upon our senses and register upon our minds.

The newspapers, radio and television all have a tremendous influence on our thought processes and mental outlook. If we carefully analyze the main news headlines in the media, we find that the greatest atrocities of the day are highlighted. The most recent incidents of murder, violence, political conflict, war, bloodshed, environmental disasters, legal battles and controversial issues are prominently highlighted, and described in the most vivid detail. Exposure to this negativity and sensationalism day after day will subliminally create a negative and depressed mental state and outlook.

The constant negative news of the daily press can cause us to lose sight of the positive side of life and positive events occurring in society. It is critical therefore for us to sometimes shut our minds off from the media and protect our thought atmosphere from the constant negativity. To initiate original thoughts and ideas, we need an opportunity to think freely, away from the constant force of external distractions. Quiet time for reflection, introspection and contemplation has always led (and will always lead) to highest quality of thoughts and ideas.

A quiet surrounding is essential for original thought. The highest and noblest ideas will surface in these moments of calm and quiet. We need moments of solitude when we must get away from the crowd. We must not go to the extent where we become a recluse, but we need to take time away from the hustle and bustle of daily existence. This can take the form of a walk in a wide spacious field, a trip to the hills or mountainside or retreating to a private room or designated area where we are able to rest, reflect and free ourselves from all distractions.

Our private areas must allow us to retire from our normal hectic activities. Periods of time must be spent here alone, in peace and quiet. Through calming of the mind, freeing ourselves from worry and hurry, and even developing the art of meditation, new ideas will manifest themselves, and a new state of well being and peace will be achieved. During meditation, we learn to free our mind from thoughts which are flowing hither and thither and which lack force and power. We develop the art of listening to our innermost mental state, being receptive to our subconscious realm. From the depths of our being new ideas will flow, full of force and vitality, generating new enthusiasm and motivation for success. In these states, we achieve a glimpse of the Positive Spirit.

To realize our goals, it is essential that we develop and nurture the art of creative visualization. In the age of innocence, when we were children, our imagination and powers of visualization were vibrant, alive and uninhibited. As we grew older and became mature, we learnt to think logically, analytically and within the normal boundaries and conventions of society. We gradually lost the full power and potency of the power of imagination. We need to return to the state of creative visualization and imagination as the starting point for awakening the Positive Spirit and achieving our dreams.

With creative visualization, we must first express desire for the goals we want to achieve. After this step, we must free our mind from doubt and believe in our ability to achieve what we desire. This is a critical step, and a lack of understanding has caused the downfall of many people. Most individuals are able to visualize what they want, but do not believe in their ability to achieve their goals. The lack of self-confidence and the belief that success and happiness are elusive goals, perpetually out of reach, causes a lack of accomplishment. Once we acquire self-confidence, and truly believe in ourselves, we can successfully materialize our desires.

One of the most critical factors for success is strong belief in ourselves and in our personal ability. History is rich with examples of great personalities who possessed faith and belief in themselves, and were able to conquer the world. We must realize our unlimited power. Anything our mind can conceive, and truly believe, it can achieve. We are what we think we are, for as the saying goes 'As a man thinketh, so shall he be.' Belief is vital for success. If we do not believe in ourselves, how can we expect others to believe in us? Lack of self confidence will only inhibit our progress.

Doubt in ourselves is the root cause of failure. Faith in ourselves, in our ability to accomplish our personal hopes, dreams and desires is the cornerstone of our success. Once we possess belief, we must take positive action towards achieving the goals we desire, and possess the will power to persist until we realize our dreams. We can overcome all obstacles in our path once we believe in ourselves and have the will power to carry on. The greatest achievements of science, technology, art, music, literature and philosophy have been the products of concentrated thought, personal belief and action. These achievements are manifestations of the Positive Spirit.

The world around us is in a constant state of evolution and change. A study of nature highlights the law of growth and progress. The plant and animal kingdom continuously experience the cycle of birth, growth and development. Similarly, mankind also experiences this continuous cycle of change. We are constantly evolving and advancing to higher states of awareness whether we are aware of it consciously or unconsciously.

As each century unfolds, new discoveries are made and new concepts are presented. In each age, understanding of the universe appears to be in an embryonic stage. Within each century are new laws, theories and concepts waiting to be unveiled. As we achieve higher states of development, physically and mentally, we unearth new insights and discoveries into the nature of the universe and the purpose of our existence.

The laws of nature expressed throughout the universe demonstrate opulence, abundance and wealth. As part of the universe, it is our right to enjoy wealth, health and happiness.

Nature always expresses and manifests itself in abundance, why should we limit ourselves and fail to enjoy that which is rightfully ours? It is our right to experience unlimited realization of our dreams and positive expressions of our goals and desires.

Constructive thinking and a positive outlook are the natural laws of the universe. Nature is a positive expression of the vital energy flow of the universe. Our ability to realize our goals and dreams will be based on our ability to clearly visualize what we desire, and to positively affirm and assert our right to achieve these desires. Realization of these goals will be based on a manifestation of the laws of nature, and the power of the positive spirit.

We must never allow mental stagnation to occur, as this will limit our progress and advancement in life. Mental stagnation strangles clear thinking, inhibiting us from realizing our full potential. Health, wealth and happiness are rightfully ours, and will be achieved through correct thought processes and mental dynamics.

The potential for greatness lies within all of us. We must be full of faith, hope and belief in our rightful claim to success. We can achieve the highest goals that we can intelligently conceive, based on belief in ourselves. Even when we make mistakes, these must serve as lessons for improvement. With positive mental attitude, constructive thinking and belief in ourselves, we are destined for success and unleashing the full power of the Positive Spirit.

# 8

# THE DIVINE SPIRIT

Man is a multi-dimensional being, consisting of the physical, mental and spiritual dimensions. The level of development of each dimension depends on the personal experiences, outlook and philosophy of each individual. Our understanding and awareness of these dimensions evolves as we progress through life.

In our lowest level of development, our existence and awareness is mainly in the physical realm. In this stage, we focus mainly on eating, drinking, sleeping and sensual activity. We are unaware of the higher stages of life, and of the greater purpose of existence. At this stage of development, we are just above the state of the animal realm. Our raw energy and passions drive our daily existence.

It has been postulated by many philosophers, that by our very nature, we are prone to evil and wrongdoing. It has been proposed that without rules, laws, checks and balances we would tend to do wrong, if we could get away with it. For example, if we could withdraw large sums of money from the bank, which did not belong to us, without being caught, how many of us would truly resist the temptation? Without the threat of criminal prosecution, how many of us would refrain from any wrongdoing? If it is innate in us to do wrong, we are at the base physical stage of existence.

As we progress in life, we enter the realm of the moral dimension. Morality represents the characteristic within us to do that which is good and accepted as right action. In this state, we recognize our innate weakness and work to improve ourselves and practice upright behaviour. We strive to develop ourselves and practice that which is noble and honourable. Our intentions are good, but sometimes we may falter and perform wrong actions.

In the moral dimension, unlike in the physical state, we are bothered when we do that which is wrong. These actions rest heavily on our conscience. We resemble the baby that is trying to walk, but stumbles after a few steps. The intentions are good, but the actions can lead to our downfall. Like the child, we will persist in our attempts to walk until we can stand on our two feet.

As we progress and develop further, encountering new experiences and discovering wisdom and insight, we move into the enigmatic spiritual realm. We venture into a realm of abstract understanding, and discover the secrets of the Divine Spirit. We unlock new doors and walk on new pathways that we have not known before.

From the beginning of time mankind has pondered upon creation and existence. "Who am I? Where am I? What is the purpose of my existence?" These questions have provoked further thought within us and a search for understanding. "Why are we here in the world? Where are we going? How are we going to get there?" These questions continue to stir debate and discussion between philosophers of varying schools of thought and belief.

Of all the questions asked, there has been one particular question which has provoked the most discussion, disagreement, variation of opinion, thought, belief and interpretation. What was responsible for the creation of the limitless universe, cosmos, galaxies or more importantly, who? Attempts to answer this key question serve as the starting point for discovering ourselves, our true identity and unveiling our purpose and the meaning of life.

When we study the world around us, we understand the principle of cause and effect. For every painting, there was a painter. For every architectural design, there was an architect. For all beautiful music and symphony, there was a musician or composer. For every work of art, there was an artist. Can we not argue, therefore, that for the greatest work of art, the universe, there was a supreme creator, artist or architect? If this is indeed so, we must further ask ourselves, what is the nature, temperament and qualities of this Supreme force? Understanding this Supreme Being will allow us to further understand some of the esoteric concepts of life.

Human experience is the ultimate testimony of the reality or existence of any phenomena. For example, we cannot see heat, but we can physically experience this condition. When the weather is hot, or if we place our hand in a fire, we personally experience the heat. Even though we cannot physically see happiness, sadness or depression, these are qualities that we can feel and personally experience. Such is the example of the Divine Being. We cannot physically see the Supreme Creator, but we can personally experience the Divine presence. Human experience throughout the ages bears testimony of several mystical and divine experiences.

In all countries, and at all stages of society, there have been thousands of personalities of spiritual advancement appearing to serve the people. There have been eyewitness accounts, testimonies and documented incidents of spiritual enlightenment and rapture. There are books which document the revealed words of the Divine Being. Spiritual giants and phenomenal religious personalities such as Noah, Abraham, Ishmael, Isaac, Jacob, Moses, David, Solomon, Zoroaster, Buddha, Krishna, Jesus, Muhammad (Upon whom be peace), have graced the face of the earth. Their lives, their trials, their experiences, their victory against all challenges provide vivid and glorious testimony of the potency and power of the Divine Spirit.

The great religions of the world teach of the existence of a Supreme lord and master responsible for all creation. This being is described as Omnipotent, Omnipresent and Omnescient. The Supreme Being is described as the possessor of mighty attributes and power, generating love, mercy and forgiveness. The creator is described as a Being that nourishes creation from stage unto stage until it achieves perfection.

Just as a mother nourishes her offspring from an infant to a child, through the stage of youth and on to adulthood, so too is the Divine Being described as nurturing all creation. Religious scriptures describe the Master of the Universe as being Beneficent, Merciful, Mighty, Wise, Aware, Majestic, Powerful, Knowing and Supreme. The combination of these divine attributes provides a brief insight into the Holistic Being society refers to as Almighty God. This ultimate source of energy, power, potency and vitality is the Supreme creator. Introspection and self-analysis leading to this understanding opens a floodgate of knowledge and new understanding of our true nature, and the higher purpose of our existence.

If we are able to unveil and discover the existence of this Supreme Being, the next step in our evolution is to question our relationship with this supreme source of power. The scriptures of the great religions, and the lessons of prophets, teach us that the key purpose of life is to unlock our true potential, to discover the higher source of our creation, and to inculcate the higher attributes and qualities of the Divine Being into our daily lives. It is our destiny to unfold into a higher realm of spirituality, and to be of greater service and value to our fellow men and society.

The attributes of the Divine Being are qualities for us to develop. We must colour ourselves with the attributes of the Supreme source of power and sustenance, Almighty God. The Supreme Being radiates love and mercy; we must also generate and radiate love and mercy. The Supreme Being is mighty and wise; we must also be mighty and wise in our affairs and dealing with our fellow men. God demonstrates forgiveness to all creation; we must also demonstrate forgiveness to those around us.

We must all be aware of our infinite potential and power for advancement and progress. Within all of us is the ability to conquer challenges, achieve our goals, and realize our hopes, dreams and aspirations. We must not view ourselves as hopeless mortals, but as children of the Supreme Being, possessing higher qualities of spirituality and consciousness. We must see ourselves as Spiritual giants, walking the face of the earth. Through introspection, self analysis, correct action and service to humanity, we gain awareness of the Divine Spirit within us. We must understand that we are higher than mere physical forces, but possess a reservoir of infinite ethereal power unknown to many of us. We are intimately connected to the Divine Being, each one of us possessing the Divine spirit.

Throughout the ages, many have looked outward in the universe in search of the Divine Spirit. This search led men to worship the sun, the moon, stars and other celestial bodies as Gods. In ancient literature, there are many reports and stories of King Solomon. In one of these accounts, there is the description of one of the opulent palaces of King Solomon, within which was a floor made of glass. Under this floor of glass, was a clear stream of water flowing. An individual walking on this floor could not tell the difference between the floor, and running water, and would literally believe that they were walking on water.

King Solomon used this room to create a deliberate illusion for his subjects and guests, to teach them an important lesson of philosophy. An individual may walk on glass, and mistake it for water. Similarly, we may witness the creation of God, and mistake it for the creator. The sun, moon, stars and other elements of nature are the Created, and not the Creator. These objects are only signs of a higher force, a higher source of energy and power responsible for what we see in nature.

We need to change our focus in our search for the Divine Being. Instead of looking outward, we must first look inward. In striving to understand our purpose, we must first seek to know ourselves. We must know our strengths and our weaknesses, and develop strategies for self-development and growth. When we look within, we will discover the power of Divinity. We discover the power to love, to care, to show mercy, compassion, courage and forgiveness. We will discover the power to become the highest, the noblest and the most sublime. These are manifestations of our Divinity and inherent greatness. Once we gain this awareness, we open the floodgates of knowledge and wisdom, and are on the highest path of development.

Having gained insight on our temperament, we will develop new focus, vision and purpose. We will walk in the path of Divine light and knowledge. This world, all our experiences within it, will be the stepping stone to a higher plane of existence. We will transcend the realm of physical actions and experience, into the highest planes of spirituality and enlightenment.

When we study our universe, we witness perfect order, harmony and precision. The laws of nature are exact and systematic. When we review the last one hundred years of human existence, we observe significant scientific, technological advancement and progress with a greater understanding of the laws of the universe. We realize how engrossed society becomes with material advancement and accomplishment. Our egos become inflated and we believe that we are the true masters of the universe, unconnected to any higher source or form. We begin to deny the existence of any higher source of power.

The events prior to December 31, 1999 bear testimony to our need for humility and greater understanding of our true nature. The uncertainty, fear and doubt we faced based on the Y2K challenge highlighted our limitations and weakness. The actual oversight in computer programming responsible for the problem, and billions of US dollars in economic loss and reprogramming cost exposed our lack of vision and foresight. We were humbled as a civilization with the Y2K experience. Our potential to make mistakes, and our inferior status in the universe was unveiled. We must learn from this lesson about the true source of all power and energy.

In the realm of creation, mankind is the highest created being in the universe. We must not forget the difference between the Creator and the Created. We may be the highest form of creation in this world, with all the forces of nature subservient to us, but the Divine being is the ultimate force of the entire universe, the Supreme Creator responsible for all existence. When we think of the word universe, we realize that it can be divided into two syllables, 'uni' and 'verse'. 'Uni' refers to oneness, and 'verse' refers to song. The meaning of universe can be described as one song, one vibration, one frequency throughout all of creation, and that is the vibration of the Divine Being,

Science teaches us about the continuous vibration of atoms, the building blocks of the universe. Matter is never still, it is very dynamic, in continuous motion. A table may appear to be static, but within the substructure are atoms in continuous motion. The solid, liquid and gaseous states are manifestations of different levels of atomic vibration. Water can exist as ice, liquid or steam based on variations in temperature and pressure, impacting upon the total atomic vibration. This change in state and form is similar to our level of spiritual development. Each and every one of us possesses latent spirituality, which is vibrating at different levels, generating varying energy levels.

We all possess an intimate link and connection with the Divine source, the true master and creator of the universe. We need to look within to discover our potentiality, our greatness, our true destiny. Through our own self analysis, we will discover the Divine Spirit. This state represents the highest state of purity and goodness that exists within all of us. Achieving this state will allow us to understand the purpose of our existence, our relationship with our fellow human beings, and out true role in society. This is the highest expression of the Spirit of Youth.

# ENHANCING THE SPIRIT

# 9

# THE POWER OF BELIEF

Having discovered the different aspects of the spirit, how do we realize our real potential? How do we effectively unlock our creative energy and power? We all have different hopes, dreams and aspirations in life. What makes the difference between continually achieving these dreams, or failing to do so? What separates those who always accomplish specified goals compared to those who are unable to do so? The answer to these questions makes the difference between success and failure in our endeavours.

As we seek to understand ourselves, and unveil our true purpose, we must first ask the question, 'What is the major obstacle and limitation to our progress in life?' After careful analysis and evaluation, we will realize that the major downfall in most of us is a lack of confidence in ourselves. We doubt our ability and question our potential for success. We hesitate when opportunities arise, fearful that we will make mistakes. This self-doubt, hesitation and low self-esteem bar the way to unlimited progress. At times, we are our worst enemies.

To truly achieve success in life, to realize our personal goals and aspirations, we must firmly believe in ourselves. We must be assertive, confident and undaunted by tasks before us. We must exude an aura of cool, calm and composure as we realize that unlimited success is our birthright. We have nothing to be fearful of, as we have all the resources required to achieve any goal that we desire. We must belief in our ability to be successful. If we do not believe in ourselves, and doubt our own ability, how do we expect others to believe in us? Belief is the essential ingredient in unlocking our potential for accomplishing our dreams.

The human mind has tremendous power to shape, mould and create the future. Our thoughts are mental vibrations which become manifested in the physical world. The creative energy, power and force of our thoughts impact on our immediate environment and surroundings. Our level of accomplishment is directly linked to our thoughts and mental activity.

It is through personal belief that some of the greatest achievements of society have been realized. A study of the lives of great personalities throughout history highlights a common, underlying component, which is the tremendous faith and ability they possessed in their ability to realize their dreams. This belief grounded into their personal character, and propelled them to the greatest heights, separating them from the rest of society.

All of the great personalities, scientists, explorers and adventurers were ridiculed and laughed at. Their ideas were different from the accepted norms and standards of society. They dared to be different, to challenge established thoughts, customs, habits and ideas. They were not content to simply follow, but ventured boldly to lead. This brought about ridicule and even retribution from the society that they challenged.

Scientists such as Aristotle, Galileo, Sir Isaac Newton and Albert Einstein dared to challenge the orthodox thinking of society. Their personal thoughts, ideas and beliefs have revolutionized the world we live in, and changed our very way of life. It is their personal belief in their ability which led them to discover the secrets of the universe, and which propelled them to the pinnacle of their fields of activity.

Personal entrepreneurs and businessmen such as Henry Ford, Walt Disney, Colonel Sanders, Stephen Bechtel and Bill Gates are testimony to the power of belief in one's ideas and personal ability to achieve success. The pioneers of human civilization, the creators of new technology, the initiators of technological advancement and progress were all human beings with remarkable vision and foresight. They understood the power of belief, the volatility of personal dreams and ideas, and the drive required to make these ideas into reality.

The pioneers of civilization believed that man could fly through the air, delve deep below the sea, journey to space and discover the secrets of the universe. Through the conception of ideas, personal belief, action, determination and drive, the great achievements of society were realized. It is important for us to understand the importance of taking action, once we have an idea. Pure belief without any action will not lead to an end result. We must act upon our belief, taking action with self-confidence that the desired goal will be realized.

The door to accomplishment is still open to us. It is only for us to embrace the opportunities and walk on through. We must start to believe in ourselves and in our ability to achieve whatever we desire. We must believe in our ability to crystallize our inner most thoughts and ideas into a new reality. We must believe in our ability to positively impact on the world around us and take affirmative action to do so. Belief in ourselves is the first step in our journey towards conquest and unlimited success.

The Spirit of Youth will soar to great heights once we embrace the philosophy of belief. By working smarter, almost like magic, our dreams become a reality. Whether it is at work, school or play, we can accomplish all that we desire. Whether it is examinations, athletic competition, artistic performance, opening a new business or getting a new job, we can be successful in all of our ventures. Through belief, positive action, hard work, determination and drive, the world is our playground for creating our desires.

Visualization is one of the most powerful techniques for achieving our goals. One of the most under-utilized aspects of our minds is the power of imagination. As children, we possessed vivid imaginations, and were very creative. As we grew older, through the stages of youth and adulthood, we were trained to think more logically and systematically, and along the way loss the true ability to harness the power of imagination. Our lack of creativity is due to our being cut off from the essential mental techniques required.

We need to tap into the creative potential and power of our minds. We must use the power of visualization to unleash our creative talent and energy. What is it that we want out of life? What are our goals and aspirations? What have we accomplished to date? What do we hope to accomplish? Through the technique of visualization, we create images in our mind of the goals that we desire.

Through concentration on these images daily, we subliminally set the forces in motion to make them into reality. Concentration on mental images gives them additional momentum and fuels them with the energy required to materialize. Having established mental images, we must take action to make these goals into reality.

Every accomplishment started as a thought in the mind of an individual. By continuously concentrating on these thoughts, adding colour, sound and shape to these ideas, applying hard work, faith and coordinated effort, these thoughts will become a reality. We must not let the fear of failure inhibit us. We must develop a positive attitude towards life, firmly believing in our right to experience success and happiness.

The Twenty-first century will present us with many new and exciting challenges and opportunities. It will be a revolutionary period highlighting the power of ideas, new technology and innovation. The formula for success will be based on belief in ourselves and the willpower to turn ideas into reality. We must embrace the opportunities presented to us, overflowing with belief and confidence in our ability to conquer all that life has to offer.

# 10

## MENTAL DYNAMICS

One of the most complex, intricate and enigmatic aspects of our existence is the human mind. Many have sought to discover its secrets, few have truly succeeded. Understanding the nature of the mind is one of the most important journeys that we must undertake in our lives. Our mental processes have the power to determine the level of success or failure in our endeavours. Our thoughts create the future, and shape the world that we live in today and which we will experience tomorrow.

A critical review of the different dimensions of the mind indicates that it can be subdivided into at least two distinct levels, the conscious and subconscious levels. In the conscious mind our present thoughts and feelings are manifested. These are directly affected by our surroundings and immediate environment. The headlines in the newspaper, the programs on television, the music on the radio, the daily conversation and opinion of society all have a direct impact and impression on our conscious mind. In this state we are operating at the periphery of the real potential of the mind.

The true power and creativity of the mind lies within the subconscious realm. When trying to understand the operation of the mind, we must think of the analogy of an iceberg. We can see the tip of the iceberg, but the true power lies beneath the surface. So too is it with our mind. We can easily see the conscious level, but true power exists at the subconscious level.

Our subconscious level is responsible for all of our involuntary actions such as breathing, circulation, digestion and other major bodily functions. The subconscious mind never rests, and is at work twenty four hours a day. During the period of sleep, our conscious mind achieves rest, while the subconscious continues to ensure the efficient operation of our body. Understanding the inter-relationship between the conscious and subconscious mind will open up new insight and understanding into the treasures which are hidden within us.

The thoughts of the conscious mind permeate into the subconscious realm. Our conscious thoughts are manifestations of that which we desire. It is our subconscious mind which goes to work on making our thoughts a reality. Our conscious thoughts become instructions which the subconscious mind will implement and strive to achieve. If for example we desire material wealth, our subconscious will evaluate different opportunities and possibilities to acquire wealth. Have we ever wondered where our ideas spring forth from, or what causes them to occur? Suddenly we may get a new and exciting idea from out of nowhere. This is the result of the subconscious mind working to make thoughts into a reality.

Our thoughts within the conscious realm impact directly

on our state of well being. Negative thinking at the conscious level impacts on our subconscious, causing ill effects on our overall physical and mental states. If we are negative and depressed, our physical health and well being will be severely compromised. Modern science has shown that the majority of diseases are traced to psychosomatic issues. There is a direct relationship between the mind and the physical body, and we must strive to understand this to achieve proper health. Positive thinking impacts beneficially on our subconscious, leading to good health and radiance.

By establishing positive thoughts, visualizing our desires, and expressing belief in our ability to achieve our goals, our subconscious mind implements mechanisms to ensure that these desires are achieved. The true source and reservoir of ideas and creativity can therefore be seen as our subconscious mind. By thinking about our goals in the conscious level, our subconscious evaluates the problems, and generates ideas and suggestions for accomplishing our dreams. This is the realm from which all new ideas spring forth.

Our personal attitude is important to our state of mental well being. If we possess a negative attitude, and always have a negative outlook in life, we cannot attract success. If mentally we dwell upon failure, then failure will become a way of life. If we develop a positive attitude, and positive state of thinking, then we attract positive events to our lives. We become highly energized and magnetized and attract whatever we truly desire.

Our thoughts are critical in determining our level of personal success. Mental dynamics, our thought processes, impact on the level of achievement we realize in life. It is essential that we develop proper mental dynamics and eliminate inhibitors from our lives. It is essential that we eliminate mental poisons which slow us down, erode our good health, and prevent us from achieving the goals that we desire. Poor mental habits eventually cause depression and disorientation, and in severe cases can lead to suicide. What are some of the mental poisons which we must strive to eliminate? What are these poisons which wreck havoc and cause unwanted destruction to proper mental dynamics and thought patterns? A careful analysis and review of the key factors which impact negatively on our mental realm is the first step towards resolving the issues and challenges caused by poor thought patterns.

Doubt is the first inhibitor to human advancement and progress. Doubt in our personal ability limits our success. Self doubt, questioning our personal ability and lack of self confidence prevent us from moving forward and achieving our goals. Self doubt creates a very negative impression on our mind. Harbouring doubtful thoughts in the conscious realm inhibits the subconscious from generating opportunities to move forward and causes inaction.

Another key inhibitor to progress is fear. Fear is one of the most crippling and limiting forces existing within the universe. Fear of criticism, fear of failure, fear of those in authority, fear of ill health, fear of financial problems and fear of life itself all lead to lack of accomplishment and lack of success. The mind attracts that which it dwells upon. The more we succumb to fear and dwell on negative thoughts, the more energy we provide to these thoughts and cause them to become a reality.

All thoughts, positive or negative, when fueled with enough energy, focus and attention will become a reality. Do we really want to crystallize negative thoughts? I think not. We need to eliminate fear and focus on the positive. The opposite of fear is faith. In fact, all negatives can be replaced by their positives. We need to inculcate more positive expectations and energy in our lives and acquire faith. Through faith, hope and positive thinking we can achieve unlimited success in all of our undertakings.

Worry is another inhibitor to progress. Worry tears to pieces the structures we have built within the mental realm. Like a wrecking ball slamming into a building, worry destroys our plans and creations. We worry about our health, wealth, family, jobs, finances, children, education and many other factors. It is important to express concern for what is happening in our lives, but worry will destroy our physical, mental and spiritual well-being. Worry is a precursor to stress and the combined effect is total havoc on the body.

The majority of people in society complain about stress due to the pressures of daily life. Whether it is at work or school, people complain about the devastating impact of stress. Scientifically, stress is referred to as pressure or tension exerted on an object. This causes a demand on energy. This description vividly describes the net forces and power of stress in our daily lives, the sensation of force or pressure being exerted upon us. We need to understand the causes of stress, its effects, and measures to significantly reduce these causes of personal stress.

What exactly causes stress? Is it the pressures at work, school or home? Is it due to family problems, financial issues or concern for our personal health and our loved ones? Is it due to the dissatisfaction with our lives, lack of achievement, or poor personal performance? We need to determine the root cause and develop measures to deal with stress.

A major cause of stress is our attitude to the challenges we face in life. We all face many challenges and will continuously face trials and tribulations which test us. It is our personal attitude and outlook when faced with these major challenges which determines the level of stress we create. Life is not about what happens to us, it is how we deal with what happens to us. If we lose our job, fail an examination, have financial difficulty, it is our attitude toward the situation which will determine how successful we are in overcoming it or how stressed out we become.

Someone who loses their job can go into a serious bout of depression, feeling a low sense of self-esteem and feeling like a complete failure in life. Another person will carefully assess the situation as an opportunity to explore a new career path, to do something which they always wanted to do, like starting their own business. A different individual may become even suicidal, while someone else will be thankful for the gift of life, the gift of health and strength to face the challenges of a new day. The person may have lost their job, but they may still have good health and strength. They still have the ability to think, to create and shape ideas, concepts and beliefs. All is not lost. Where there is life, there is hope. It is therefore the outlook on the situation which dictates the level of stress, and not the situation itself.

Our physical and mental processes can become out of control due to fear, worry and stress. Because of stress our muscles tighten, our bowels loosen, sweat flows, adrenalin pumps, our breathing becomes fast and shallow with the physical body entering a state of turmoil. We will feel intense mental pressure, like an invisible force pressing down upon us. We must eliminate fear and worry and take control of our body. Concern for life is important, but fear, worry and panic will wreck havoc and cause utter chaos.

Our mental dynamics are an integral part of our existence.

Good mental dynamics will determine health, strength and emotional well-being. We need to calm the mind, and become cool and composed. We live in a world of tremendous uncertainty, and must be prepared for the unexpected. We need to go on a mental diet and control the thoughts we let into our system. We must eliminate negative thoughts and expectations from our mind. With a proper mental diet, we will realign our thinking and take control of our emotional well being and future happiness.

True success in life does not depend on what happens to us, but how we deal with what happens to us. We need to apply wisdom to the daily occurrences in our lives, and believe that everything happens for a purpose. There is meaning in the events around us, and we must derive the lessons from these experiences. How we deal with the challenges of daily life and our personal attitude to these challenges will determine our level of success or personal failure.

By understanding the fluid nature of mental dynamics, the operation of the mind, and the inter-relationship between the conscious and sub-conscious realm, the Spirit of Youth will be enhanced and prepared for the challenges of the future. By implementing positive mental habits, thought processes and activity, the Spirit of Youth will unlock our inner power and creativity leading to the fulfillment of our personal hopes, dreams and aspirations.

# 11

## OUR INFINITE POTENTIAL

Who am I? Where am I? What is the purpose of my existence? These are immortal questions which have provoked the mind of man since the beginning of time. It is this search for understanding throughout the ages which has generated the diversity of opinions, theories and beliefs on the purpose of our existence. Many great personalities who walked the face of the earth left for us their personal philosophy, teachings and writings on achieving meaning out of life.

With the dawn of the New Millennium, the search for understanding will continue. New ideologies, philosophies and concepts will be presented. New discoveries will be made which will shed greater light on the complexity of human nature. The questions we will continue to ask include, "What is our true potential? What is the highest level of achievement that the human spirit can achieve in the different spheres of life?" In attempting to answer these probing questions, we will gain further insight into our true self.

As we look at the society around us, we realize that everyone is aspiring to achieve success in their personal sphere of activity. Different people have different definitions of success based on their personal goals, values and belief systems. Some measure success by the acquisition of knowledge, others by the accumulation of wealth, the achievement of power or prominent status in society. To measure their perceptions of success in society people use different benchmarks.

Whatever our definition of success, how can it be achieved? What is necessary for an individual to be successful in life? Further to this, what separates those who have achieved success from those who have not? A careful analysis of the situation indicates that personal belief in one's ability is the critical ingredient necessary for success. The self-made millionaire, the prosperous young professional, the skilled tradesman, all have belief in their personal skills and ability to achieve success in all their efforts. This positive attitude and mental outlook separates these individuals from the rest of society.

Underachievement in society is closely linked to lack of personal belief and low self-confidence. The reasons why many people struggle for daily existence, barely coping with the daily pressures of life, are linked to low self esteem and a negative attitude to life. Many of us become very disoriented and disenchanted when obstacles appear in our lives. When faced with challenges, we may become depressed and pessimistic. Our personal attitude to obstacles and perceived problems will determine our level of advancement and progress.

The word 'problem' plays a significant role in limiting our advancement in life. When a situation develops which we consider a 'problem', we feel limited in our ability to move forward. We need to eliminate the word 'problem' from our vocabulary and replace it with the word 'challenge'. We should not think in terms of 'problems', but instead think of these situations as 'challenges' which we have the potential to overcome. We should use these 'challenges' as learning experiences for our personal development and maturity.

If we could accomplish anything we desire, what would it be? What are our personal goals or dreams? What is it that we have always wanted to achieve and have never gotten around to doing? We should sit and contemplate our lives, reflect upon what it is that we have always desired. After we have done this, we must ask ourselves, 'Why have we not accomplished our dreams, and what has prevented us from doing so?' The answer to this question, most of the time, is lack of confidence in ourselves and fear of failure.

Every one of us has the potential to achieve our dreams, but it is our lack of belief, our negative attitude and poor mental dynamics which inhibits us from realizing grand achievements. We possess infinite potential to achieve any goal that we desire. The key to realizing this potential is developing proper thought processes and personal attitude to situations. Through positive attitude and belief systems, we will chart a guaranteed course to success.

Human nature is an intricate blend of the Physical, Mental and Spiritual dimensions. Our individual perception and understanding of ourselves will determine our personal evolution and unfolding. Those who view themselves as merely a physical being limit their true potential. At the physical stage, we resemble the animals that eat, sleep and pro-create via instinct. If we do not understand our higher levels of existence, we are unable to really move forward.

Greater understanding and awareness of the mental dimension opens a whole new vista for transcendence. Understanding the tremendous potency and vitality of our mental faculties will unveil pathways to unlimited success in life. Proper understanding of our conscious and unconscious minds, with a proper understanding of the creative power of visualization and imagination, will make us realize success effortlessly. Proper understanding of will power, concentration and the need for mental discipline will make us masters over our destiny.

As we gain understanding and awareness of our physical and mental states, we will become aware of even higher dimensions. This will lead us onto the path of the Spiritual dimension. As we move upward from the realm of the physical into the spiritual dimension, we enter a new kingdom and domain of knowledge which transcends the ordinary states of existence. We enter the gateway of infinite accomplishment and self-realization.

A review of religious philosophy throughout the ages highlights underlying similarities and common messages on the true essence of human nature. All religious scriptures highlight the infinite power, potency and potential of mankind. The immortal and transcendent nature of human beings is given utmost focus and significance in all religious teachings.

Hinduism highlights the infinite power and potential of the human spirit in the scriptures of the Bhagavad Gita and the Vedas. The techniques for achieving harmony and union of the physical, mental and spiritual states are taught via yoga and other ancient techniques. The infinite nature of our existence is presented in the Bhagavad Gita in Chapter 2, Verses 23-24:

*'The soul can never be cut to pieces by any weapon, nor burned by fire, nor moistened by water, nor withered by the wind.*

*The individual soul is unbreakable and insoluble, and can be neither burned nor dried. He is everlasting, present everywhere, unchangeable, immovable and eternally the same.'*

Christianity also teaches the immortality of mankind. Within the pages of the Holy Bible, there are many references on the infinite power of mankind as presented in Psalms 82:6:

*'I have said that Ye are Gods; and all of you are children of the most High'*

Judaism highlights the high levels of spirituality which can be achieved by mankind, as demonstrated by the greatness of prophets of Israel such as Moses, David and Solomon. The great prophet – kings of Israel such as David and Solomon achieved an unparalleled combination of spiritual, moral and material greatness. They combined spirituality with vast material riches and opulence.

Islam teaches that mankind was created as a ruler or God's representative on earth. The Arabic word Khalifa is used to describe mankind, which means ruler, king or master. The teachings of the Holy Prophet Muhammad (uwbp) highlight the importance of understanding our true nature, and focus on developing our moral and spiritual values.

In the Holy Qur'an Chapter 2 Verse 20 it states:

*'And thy Lord said to the angels*

*I am going to place a ruler in the earth'*

The teachings of Buddhism highlight the need for mankind to understand their infinite spiritual power and potential. Just as a bee is restless until it finds comfort in the nectar of the flower, so too must mankind seek to find comfort in the nectar of spiritual bliss. In addition to these religions highlighted, a review of other religions highlights similar concepts and teachings on the means to spiritual awakening, advancement and enlightenment.

The greatest religious philosophies and ideologies have represented mankind as immortal beings walking the face of the earth. Our journey through life is a process of realizing our true nature and unlocking our infinite potential. We are limited in life when we think of ourselves in limited terms. When we view ourselves as poor, helpless, mortal beings, we are unable to realize our infinite potential.

Religious scriptures teach that the world is a temporary plane of existence and is a stepping stone to a higher stage of life. Our real purpose is to return to our pure state of spiritual energy and vitality. We must elevate ourselves continuously. We must evolve from the physical state into the moral and pristine realm of spirituality.

Every one of us possesses a spark of infinity deep within. When we realize our essence only then can we aspire to release our infinite potential. Only then can the dreams that we desire become a reality. When we achieve insight and understanding of our true nature, the enlightenment will allow us to walk the path of success.

Through introspection, meditation and fearless action, we will unlock our latent power. When we sit in quiet surroundings and aim to calm the mind, we gain a greater awareness of our true self. The mind is restless and in continuous motion. In a state of mental agitation, our breathing becomes fast and shallow. Through slow, deep breathing, we can have a calming effect on the mind. When we calm the mind, it becomes peaceful and serene like the surface of a lake. If we throw pebbles in the lake, ripples appear disturbing the peaceful surface. Such is the case with mental agitation which causes ripples and waves through the mind.

When we achieve inner peace, calm and quiet through

meditation, we can gain awareness of our higher states. As we sit quietly, thoughts come forth from deep within our sub-conscious, revealing our true energy and vitality. We are able to discover ourselves. We gain awareness of our true purpose. We gain awareness of an infinitely higher presence dwelling within us. This state is significantly higher than our physical state and represents a glimpse of our Infinite potential. This self- realization is an essential stepping stone to realizing our goals in life.

# 12

# ACHIEVING OUR GOALS

Goals are our guiding light as we journey through life, giving us direction, focus and meaning. To accomplish all of our desired tasks, we must have well-defined goals and targets. If we do not know where we are going, how do we plan to get there? If we do not know where we are going, then any road will do. Without proper direction or guidance, we will be unable to reach a meaningful destination.

Every one of us has different hopes, dreams and aspirations. Through proper belief systems, planning and determination, these dreams can become a reality. In working to accomplish our tasks, we must implement a systematic approach. First of all, we must clearly define our present position, status and circumstances in life. What are our personal strengths? What are our areas of weakness? Secondly, we must define our goals and aspirations. Thirdly, we must develop a strategic plan to accomplish these desires. Fourthly, we must take action to achieve our goals and be prepared for unplanned events or obstacles which may not have been considered originally.

The process of working toward accomplishment of goals can be summarized by asking ourselves the following questions: "Where am I in life? Where would I like to be? How do I plan to get there?" Through introspection and self analysis we can establish our present status and develop plans and projections for further advancement.

To achieve success in life, we must have clearly defined goals. We must however believe in our ability to achieve these goals, and take action to do so. We can look at the example of a college student to gain further insight on this subject. To be successful in examinations, a specific course of action is required. First of all, the student must attend classes to receive the necessary tuition from teachers. If some classes are missed, the student must obtain these notes from fellow classmates. A review of the syllabus of the specific courses must be carried out. A proper study program and review of textbooks, notes and research material must also be performed.

Further to these requirements, the student must do past paper questions for the different courses. Effective time management techniques must be developed for studies as well as for the examinations themselves. Passing examinations and achieving academic success can only be achieved through hard work, proper study techniques, commitment, dedication and determination. By setting specific goals and adopting a pragmatic approach to achieving these goals, success will be realized.

Several components are required when working to achieve our goals. Wee must visualize what we want out of life, and believe in our ability to accomplish our desires. Proper planning, focus, concentration and determination are required in our endeavours. We must take action to make our dreams into reality. Merely visualizing, wishing and hoping for something to happen without initiating action will doom us to failure and disappointment.

Perseverance in the face of perceived failure is essential. We must not become easily disenchanted, disheartened and de-motivated when things do not go our way, or when we face stiff challenges or obstacles in our path. We must be persistent until we are successful. We must demonstrate the determination to carry on no matter how dismal things may appear. This 'Never Say Die' attitude will reap unlimited rewards in life.

Strategic planning and thinking are essential ingredients in a recipe for success in life. In specifying goals, these must be further sub-divided into short term, medium term and long term goals. Short term goals can be specified as those which we strive to accomplish within one (1) year. Medium term goals can be specified as those which we want to accomplish within two to five (2-5) years. Long term goals can be specified as those which will take us more than five (5) years to accomplish. By adopting this approach, we gain a realistic insight on the duration of time required for different goals and we can plan accordingly.

An example of striving to achieve goals can be seen in the athlete preparing for the Olympic games. The athletic program will require specific short, medium and long term goals for different stages of development. A detailed program of physical training will be required. Proper diet and nutrition are essential for holistic development. An intense program facilitating well-rounded physical, mental and spiritual development will be implemented. Self motivation, discipline, focus, belief and determination are required as the athlete prepares for competition. Specific actions are required if the individual wants to achieve the desired goal and results.

We must not set mediocre goals which can easily be achieved. We must always stretch ourselves and go to new limits. We must let our imagination and creativity roam freely, and set goals of extremely high standards. We have the potential to achieve excellence, and we should never aim for less. Based on our personal beliefs, needs and temperament, our individual goals may vary, but our approach to achieving these goals must be the same.

We must be either tactical or strategic as we work to accomplish our desired goals. The example of football (soccer) can be used to illustrate the different approaches to accomplishing our targets. A tactical move occurs when the forward player (striker) gets a spontaneous opportunity and kicks the ball into the goal and scores. The strategic approach takes a little more time, and occurs when the defender passes the ball to the midfielder, who passes it to the wing player, who crosses it toward the striker who takes the shot at goal and scores. The build up is gradual, slower and more calculated but the end result is the same.

As can be seen from the example, a tactical move is a short term, direct approach to achieving what is desired. The strategic approach entails a systematic build-up as each step brings us closer to accomplishing that which is desired. The approach and techniques vary significantly, but the final result is the same. Depending on the situation and the prevailing circumstances, we can determine if a tactical or strategic approach is required.

We must be assertive and self confident as we work to achieve our goals. We must have faith in our personal ability to make our dreams a reality. Sometimes we may face challenges which initially prevent us from accomplishing our goals. Our attitude towards these challenges will determine if we fail or if we succeed. We must always be prepared for challenges, and possess the determination and will power to conquer all obstacles which appear before us.

If our goal is to become a successfully published writer, for example, we must not give up if the first few publishers we submit our manuscript to turns us down. Did we send our manuscript to the right type of publisher? Is there a similar book already written on the subject? Does our grammar require improvement? We can re-assess our initial submission, make the necessary improvements, and re-submit to another publisher. It is only through persistence and continuous struggle can we fully reap the reward of our efforts. We must try until we succeed. History bears testimony to numerous people whose ideas were initially rejected, but who later went on to make these ideas a phenomenal success.

If we want to represent our country at athletics, would we give up if we fail to qualify at the first national try-outs that we participate in? Did we train hard enough? Was something wrong with our technique? Was our diet appropriate? Do we need to get a better coach? We need to analyze our weaknesses and shortcomings and develop strategies to convert them into strengths.

Periods of failure in our lives provide fertile ground for sowing the seeds of success. Failure serves as a stepping stone to success. It provides us with valuable opportunities to re-assess our lives and develop new ideas and approaches to what we are doing. In fact, some of the greatest opportunities for unlimited success present themselves to us after we assess incidents of failure in our search for doing things better. We must learn from our mistakes and continually work to improve ourselves.

In working to achieve our goals we must be able to multi-task. Life is a dynamic process and we are always aiming to achieve many goals at the same time. We must be able to manage ourselves efficiently as we work to accomplish these tasks simultaneously. A rating system where we prioritize tasks into High, Medium and Low priority must be developed. The level of importance of each will determine the amount of time and energy we spend on working towards the different goals.

Effective time management is required as we work towards achieving multiple goals and targets. We cannot be spending the majority of our time on our lowest priority goals and the least amount of time on those of highest priority. A delicate balance must be achieved between the amount of time spent on tasks in relation to their level of priority. In developing this approach, we can effectively manage our time as we aim to achieve different goals within the specified time frames.

By developing a strategic approach to life, we will become more efficient at achieving our goals. At the beginning of each week, we must define our goals for the week ahead. We must evaluate our strategy and approach towards accomplishing these goals within specified time frames. At the end of the week, we must assess our actual performance in relation to our set targets and benchmarks, and determine how successful we have been at accomplishing our specifications. The ratio of goals achieved to goals specified will indicate our level of efficiency and identify areas for improvement and upgrade. By continually evaluating our progress weekly, monthly and annually we will significantly improve our overall efficiency and effectiveness.

Through introspection and self-analysis we will continually improve our individual performance. We will recognize areas of strength and weakness and will be able to develop techniques to further improve our performance. To be successful in life, we must continually define meaningful goals to give us focus, direction and purpose. It is only when we know where we are going, can we effectively develop a road map and plan to get there. It is through strategic planning, determination, personal belief and working smarter that we are firmly on the pathway to success and achieving our goals.

# 13

## ACQUISITION OF KNOWLEDGE

Man is a speculative being. To probe, question and analyze is an inherent part of our nature. From the beginning of time, we have questioned the purpose of our existence. We have studied the heavens and earth in an attempt to unlock its secrets. This speculative and inquisitive temperament has been the foundation of acquisition of knowledge throughout the ages.

The ancient Greek philosopher Socrates said that 'The unexamined life is not worth living.' This philosophic overture, this spirit of examining, questioning and analyzing has transcended the centuries through the work of philosophers, scientists and artists. Through their works society has acquired a wealth of knowledge in the various fields of science, art and humanities.

With the evolution of ideas and concepts, the seventeenth century French philosopher Rene Descartes asked the question, 'Is there anything of which I can be certain?' With this approach to challenging accepted beliefs, and seeking to prove and validate normally accepted theories, mankind ventured unto a new path of advancement. Through his introspection and contemplation, Descartes was able to verify one particular fact, when he was able to say with certainty 'I think.' To prove that he could think was clear validation of a particular fact. To even doubt the fact that he could think was to provide conclusive evidence of thought, as doubt itself was thought, proving the concept 'I think therefore I am'. With this illumination and starting point for analysis, numerous uncertainties were unfolded and supported with conclusive fact.

The methods of acquisition of knowledge have varied throughout history. But the philosopher may ask us, 'What exactly is knowledge?' Knowledge is an understanding, awareness or mastery of a particular field of study. It is a theoretical or practical understanding of a subject. Society has achieved significant advancement and progress through the acquisition of knowledge. The advances in science, technology, art, literature, politics, philosophy and economics have all been achieved by the continuous search and thirst for knowledge.

How do we acquire knowledge? It is through systematic questioning, probing and analysis we find ourselves on the different paths of knowledge in our particular fields of interest. The first path towards acquisition of knowledge lies in the field of formal education. Through primary, secondary and tertiary institutions, structured courses of study allow for the transfer of knowledge from teacher to student. Through these institutions of learning, students can acquire detailed knowledge on diverse subject areas.

The methods of transfer of knowledge have evolved throughout the ages. From the verbal word passed on from generation to generation, to the written word, methods have changed over the centuries. Thousands of years ago methods included hieroglyphics, code, ancient languages written on scrolls, caves, wood, bone or any available medium. With the invention of paper, and the printing press, books were able to capture the writings of our forefathers. The invention of the printing press revolutionized the mechanism of capturing human thought and ideas, making them accessible for all generations.

Within the last decade of the twentieth century, computers have revolutionized our ability to store and transfer information, allowing us to achieve greater speeds and efficiency in the transfer of information. We are evolving into a paperless society, with information being stored in cyberspace via internet technology. The internet has revolutionized our means of acquiring information and our ability to communicate across the continents. The entire world is wired and connected as one global village. Schools, universities have become 'virtual' institutions, with an increased number of Distance learning modules available for students. With the aid of a computer, and internet access, the world of information is available to us at our fingertips.

The revolution in information technology will continue to impact profoundly on our acquisition of knowledge in the twenty-first century. Further developments will provide greater tools and techniques for students to master their chosen field of study. We must proceed cautiously, however, and realize that there is a difference between the acquisition of information and the acquisition of knowledge. The volume of data available on the internet is mainly information and not knowledge. True knowledge comes from detailed understanding of a particular topic and we must be able to distinguish between raw information and crystallized knowledge.

The second path to the acquisition of knowledge is through experience. After we leave formal schooling and education, there are many valuable lessons we learn which are taught to us via practical experiences and personal encounters. This gives truth to the statement of society that 'Experience is the best teacher'. After we graduate from college or university, we enter the hectic world of work. This is a new realm of understanding in which our learning curve increases rapidly. Many of the lessons of the workplace cannot be taught in the classroom. It is only through the experience of employment that we are truly initiated into a realm of knowledge that was previously unknown.

The world of work is the making or breaking point of many young professionals. Many students would have spent their entire lives in formal institutions, with the academic realm as their only source of learning. The world of work presents challenges unlike anything ever experienced before. Some will embrace the opportunity, savour the challenge and strive to prove their self worth and ability to accomplish specified goals and targets. Others are traumatized by the aggressive environment, bruised by the graphic experiences, and yearn to return to the safety and comfort of the academic world. Survival in the workplace will depend on the individual's attitude and determination.

Many young professionals are unable to adapt to the organizations in which they gain employment. Organizational change, company restructuring, rightsizing, downsizing occurs to rapidly for them. Increased workloads, tighter deadlines, and demanding bosses create too much pressure and stress for them to cope with. The constant influx of e-mails, faxes, phone calls create increased demands on the individual to multi-task with tighter deadlines and schedules. The traditional five (5) days, forty (40) hours working week of our parents has been converted to a seven (7) day, twenty four (24) hours a day work period due to improvement in communications and computer technology. This creates anxiety and tension in the young working generation, with higher levels of stress and feelings of disenchantment and yearning for more out of life.

To other young professionals the challenges of the work place invigorates them, excites them and makes them strive to prove their superiority over the system. They never give in to the pressures of their organization and are able to overcome all challenges and obstacles. Their youth and vitality are harnessed to produce maximum results and to surpass all benchmarks and performance standards for their chosen profession.

Whatever the experiences of the young professional, the experiences of the work place is a tremendous training ground for the acquisition of knowledge. Whether it is a young tradesman out of Technical school, a University graduate in a new organization, or a young entrepreneur starting their own business, the world of work creates new experiences and allows for the acquisition of knowledge. Significant understanding of issues such as economics, organizational change, technical advancement, human resource issues, environmental policy and management principles and concepts are achieved.

One of the buzz phrases of the 1990's was 'Continuous Learning' and the need for continuous improvement. What exactly is 'Continuous Learning?' Does it only refer to the formal systematic education presented in institutions of learning? Or does it refer to continuous professional advancement gained from the experiences of the workplace and striving to learn as much as possible on our chosen field via our personal research and study? Do employers only recognize formal education, or is merit and recognition given for the practical experiences gained at work? Both forms of learning are critical, with their own benefits and advantages, and an optimum mix of both forms of learning are essential.

The third path of knowledge is based on striving to understand the true purpose of our existence. We must look within, searching to understand our true essence and seeking to unlock our unlimited potential. Mankind over the years has focussed on that which is external to him, mainly the material world and the external forces of nature. Through advancement in science and technology we have used knowledge to conquer the elements of the earth, sky and sea, even venturing into outer space and the heavens. We have developed technology to extract minerals and the riches of the earth, fly through the air and dive deep below the sea. Our technology has transformed the landscape of the regions we inhabit. The inventions of modern technology have revolutionized our standard of living.

The twentieth century witnessed an explosion of scientific discovery and technological advancement unparalleled by any other period in human existence. Having conquered the earth, we have turned our attention to the heavens. The story of the twenty first century will be the conquest of space and the outer universe. But with all of these external conquests, the question still arises, 'Do we really know who we are and where we are heading? Have we been able to conquer our inner world and understand our inner nature?' If not, we still need to acquire this vital knowledge.

In the twenty-first century, we must seek to discover our true selves. Some of us view ourselves as purely physical beings, existing in the physical realm. We think in terms of physical space because this is natural to us. Geometric space, size and quantity are very easy for us to comprehend. Others believe that we are more than physical beings, as testified by the greater dimension of the mental realm that cannot truly be quantified.

The dynamics of the mental realm unveils a whole new field of challenge for us to understand. What is the relation between the mind and the body? Which has influence or control over the other? What are the inter-relationships, and synergies between these dimensions? What are the benefits of understanding these inter-relationships? These are questions which we must seek to answer and clarify. The answers to these questions will provide enlightenment and insight into the higher purpose of our existence.

The fourth part of knowledge is based on the search for a higher dimension in man. We are aware of the physical and mental realm, but is there a higher energy or force within us known as the spiritual realm? If so, what exactly is this state of existence, and what is its relationship with the rest of the universe?

Many philosophers throughout the ages have described man as a spiritual being existing in the material world. The physical body is perceived as a vehicle for the spiritual essence, the soul, to travel in the material realm. If indeed we possess a soul, what is its nature and what is its purpose? Is it destructible? Is it eternal? Significant indeed are the implications of the answers to these burning questions.

Further questions develop as we search for answers to these initial questions. Were we created by a higher force, a primal energy that is responsible for all of creation? If so, what is the nature of this Supreme force, this Master of existence?

What is our relationship or connection with this Higher Being who is the source of all existence? Again, the implications of the answers to these questions can revolutionize personal beliefs and transform our entire outlook on the purpose of our life.

Philosophy and Religion throughout the ages have referred to a Supreme Being, a possessor of magnificent attributes responsible for all of creation. Man has been described as the vicegerent or representative of the Divine Being walking the face of the earth. Within man is the potential for greatness, for the development of lofty ideals and attributes similar to the creator. What is the pathway to unlocking these attributes? What is the path to communion and revelation from the Divine Being? Such communion or rapture will revolutionize our hearts and minds, and positively influence our relationship with our fellow human beings.

There are ancient stories of spiritual personalities who achieved revelation from the Supreme Being. These individuals experienced direct communication from the Divine. The Holy Scriptures and texts unveil messages indicating their source as the Supreme Creator and Master of the heavens of the Earth. These pages reveal a blueprint for human existence and spiritual unfolding. What lessons can we learn from these illustrious writings? What pure knowledge is locked up within these enigmatic treasure chests, waiting to be unveiled to society? The answers in these scriptures will clarify the mystery of life.

The great spiritual personalities have testified about revelation from the Divine, Spiritual Enlightenment and the existence of a Supreme Author of existence. Has revelation to mankind stopped in this modern age? Is the door to revelation and communication from the Divine closed? If not, how can we open the door to a floodgate of spiritual light and communication? How can we experience revelation from the Divine and communication in our daily lives?

Some may question the existence of such a creator. Does this Being just look passively at the problems of the earth without intervening? With global issues such as poverty, AIDS, crime, unemployment, pollution, illiteracy and racism, are there no solutions to these problems? Why does the Supreme Being not guide us or inspire us to the solution for these ills of society?

The question therefore arises, 'Will the Supreme Being contact us, or must we actively seek to contact the Divine Being?' We must first understand ourselves and our temperament, and the contribution we each have to make before we seek to understand or judge our fellow human beings. When we understand our society and global environment, only then can we truly start to understand the Divine Being and achieve support in our quest to solve key issues in society. Our search for personal answers and understanding will enlighten and inspire us to be a positive force in the quest to solve challenges of the twenty -first century.

Knowledge indeed is power. Through the acquisition of knowledge we are able to achieve understanding, inspiration and insight for the improvement of our society. Acquisition of knowledge must be a life long journey. We must seek knowledge from the cradle to the grave. The different pathways of knowledge will lead to our physical, mental and spiritual elevation and transcendence. When we actively search for the answers to the mysteries of life, we will acquire knowledge to improve the conditions of the world we inhabit. This is the master key to unlocking the reservoir of personal resources in our quest to improve the condition of society.

# 14

# THE MAGIC OF TIME

Of all the resources we possess, time is the most precious. The measure of our success as individuals is based on our ability to effectively utilize time. Life is an accumulation of events, activities and experiences, and our success is linked to our ability to effectively manage our lives within our specified allotment of time. History will judge us as to whether we were masters of time, or servants of time.

There is a direct relationship between our physical, mental and spiritual development with respect to the continuum of time. Physically, there are different stages of human development with the passage of time. These include birth, childhood, teenager/youth, adulthood, old age and eventually death. Within each phase, we undergo different levels of advancement. From the conception of a baby to birth, there are three trimesters, with each period providing its own cycle of progression and growth for the unborn child.

When we study the evolution of the universe, the development of human civilization and society, we realize that all are related to change within a specific period of time. The conquest of the material world, the ability to harness the resources of the earth, the evolution of technology are all based on human achievement and discovery within different spans of time. Many of these inventions and discoveries over the years have improved our standard of living and provided us with greater comfort and luxury.

Two key areas of improvement over the last one hundred (100) years have been in the fields of transportation and communication. Our forefathers used horses and carriages for transportation, which eventually evolved into the train and railway system. In the early twentieth century the automobile was invented establishing a new innovation in transport. From the earliest cars developed by Henry Ford, to the latest automobile models, we witness the leaps and bounds of technological advancement and improvement made with these vehicles. Cars are able to provide more reliability, efficiency and luxury for our own comfort and personal satisfaction.

We have witnessed a revolution in communications over the last few centuries. Ancient civilizations used smoke signals, falcons with messages and horsemen for communication. From the invention of the first telephone, to present day cellular technology providing video images, e-mail and text, the explosion of knowledge and scientific advancement is evident.

Satellite and GPS systems are the order of the day for personal communications. In periods of warfare, missiles and weaponry now use satellite systems to accurately pinpoint targets. When we study systems of the past, and achievements of previous generations, it prepares us for the future, and the prospective advancement we will witness in our lifetime, and which will occur in the years to come.

Genetic Engineering and other advances in medicine and health-care techniques will be at the forefront of the twenty first century. Medical research will provide us with greater understanding of the human body, with cures for disease and means to improve health and wellness. The Internet will continue to evolve, directly impacting upon all aspects of modern living including business and commerce, education, research, entertainment and general leisure. Alternate fuels will be the order of the day as we aggressively pursue means to replace the use of limited global reserves of fossil fuel.

We will achieve longer lifespans as we make advances in medicine. We will unlock further secrets of the brain and tap into previously unexplored mental realms, allowing us to better understand our neurological systems and mental dynamics. We will eventually evolve into a paperless society in the area of business transactions via e-commerce, debit/ credit cards and online systems. Society as we know it will continue to evolve, and we must adapt to the change taking place around us.

We must become masters of time, fluid thinkers who are able to hit the moving target of new events and experiences. Many of us are rigid, fixed in our general approach to life, and do not have the flexibility to quickly adapt to changes which may occur. While we are making plans, the circumstances around us will change, and we must be able to effectively deal with new challenges as they develop.

Life is a very dynamic process; it is never static. We may make plans, but things can turn out totally opposite to what we expected. We must develop the flexibility to deal with unexpected circumstances and events in our lives and manage them to our advantage. Failure to do so will cause us unprecedented stress and distress as we become constantly disoriented by unexpected events.

In every day, we each have twenty four (24) hours at our disposal. This can be further sub-divided into fourteen hundred and forty (1440) minutes or eighty six thousand, four hundred (86,400) seconds. We all have a level playing field as we are provided with the same amount of time each day. The factor that separates us into those who are successful and constantly realizing their goals and those who are not, is the ability to effectively utilize our time. Poor time management is the downfall of most of us, setting the stage for continual failure instead of unlimited success.

In any day ( 24 hour period) we all have different patterns of sleep, eating, personal hygiene, commuting to and from work / school, time spent at work / school, leisure, personal recreation, planning, reading, exercise / fitness and other miscellaneous activities. Different individuals spend varying periods of time with these activities. We witness different styles of time management in society. A significant number of people mismanage time. As soon as they get up in the morning, they are late or off-schedule and begin a frantic rush and hurry to get going. The entire day becomes a hustle and bustle trying to catch up with loss time, subliminally creating new stress and anxiety.

We must look at each day as our personal bank account with 1440 minutes (86,400 seconds). For every task we perform we must aim to save a few minutes and seconds. If we can save five (5) minutes on every hour, this translates into fourteen (14) hours a week, two (2) days a month, and a significant total of twenty four (24) days a year. We would be able to recover approximately 7% of our time annually to do whatever we desire. By saving small increments of time in simple tasks, these can accumulate to significant savings over the course of weeks and months. By breaking down the day, and trimming off the minutes and seconds from tasks, we regain control of our time.

We must have quality time to think and plan. Thoughts are the blueprints of the future. Our ideas, concepts and beliefs create the future and will revolutionize tomorrow. The pioneers of each civilization were those who spent quality time thinking, analyzing and taking action to make a difference. We must engage our mind in quiet time for thought, reflection and analysis. Powerful thoughts emanating from determined minds will reshape the world as we know it.

As a student prepares for examinations, effective study technique is essential. Appropriate time must be allocated to study each course. Knowing all the work is not the only component for examination success. Effective examination technique is vital. Students must manage their time efficiently in the examination hall to successfully complete all the exam questions. If for example, a student has one and a half (1 ½ hrs) hours to acquire 100 marks in a paper, it means that the individual must acquire approximately 1.11 marks / minute. For a question worth 20 marks, this would mean spending approximately 22 minutes on this particular question. It would be absolute chaos to spend 20 minutes on a question worth 2 marks, as this mismanagement of time will cause failure to complete the paper.

Athletes are constantly competing against the clock. In the premier event of athletics, the 100 metre race, the most acute usage of time is required. A high level of alertness, physical and mental fitness, determination and will power are essential. A nanosecond of error will cost a contender the race. The slightest margin of error makes the difference between winning the gold or silver medals. Most athletes will tell us that they did not win a silver medal, but that they lost the gold.

In the workplace, multi-tasking and the ability to deliver on schedule are critical for business success. For multiple stakeholders, we must be able to deliver on time, every time. If we were in the business of catering wedding cakes, would we have the luxury of accidentally delivering one day late? This would be impossible. One such error and our business reputation would be ruined. As the demands of the workplace continue to increase in the twenty-first century, we will be continually stretched to perform multiple tasks within schedule.

We must establish a priority matrix and criticality chart for each task we perform. Our time is precious and must be utilized accordingly. Depending on the level of importance, the level of urgency and the stakeholders involved, we can rate each task accordingly as a priority 1, 2 or 3 task, with 1 being of the highest level of importance. In our personal lives this would help us to prioritize and be more efficient in our tasks. In the work place, for example, if the Managing Director requests an assignment be completed in time for a business trip he needs to make in two (2) days, would we place the same level of priority on other work tasks which can be completed the following week? It could be career suicide to put the Managing Director's request as low priority and have it incomplete.

We must cultivate the art of patience. We live in a fast-paced society where we all want things quickly. We have fast foods, fast communications, fast cars, all of which speed up the pace at which things are delivered to us. Some of our goals will take time to accomplish. We must constantly and persistently carry on and nurture our hopes and dreams, making them into a reality. Patience and perseverance must become two of our watchwords.

If we study the art of nurturing a plant from a seed, there are many lessons that we can derive. Proper soil must be provided, weeds must be removed and the seed planted. This must be watered routinely and will eventually burst forth from the soil to bask in the sunlight. When a seed is planted in the ground, we cannot expect a giant tree to emerge in a few weeks. This requires a much longer period of time. Similarly, we must realize that certain goals will not be realized in the short term, but require much greater periods of time. With consistent effort and a systematic approach towards our personal desires, we will accomplish our goals and objectives. In addition to our efforts, we must develop the art of enjoying the journey towards our goals.

We must be able to effectively utilize time to achieve our objectives in a realistic time frame. We must be able to multi-task, plan for the unexpected, become pro-active and have more flexibility to deal with the challenges of a fast-paced society. We must be able to anticipate the future, plan effectively and use our initiative to deal with new situations and circumstances. We must lead the way for others to follow, becoming positive examples on the benefits of utilizing time effectively.

Proper time management allows us to work magic in our lives. By becoming masters of time, we can continuously achieve success in all our endeavours and positively influence society. We must treat time as a precious gift that is bestowed upon us. It must be utilized for the benefit of society, our family, friends, loved ones and ourselves. It is a waste of valuable time to perpetuate poor family relations. Conflict management and professional support should be sought to resolve family issues. Life is too short to foster ill-will and enmity within families, and such values are a very sad and negative utilization of the gift of time. It is only at the death of family members or old friends that we feel regret for all the bad relations, but at that point it is too late, as time has moved on and all we are left with are lost opportunities.

Let us use the minutes and seconds before us as the building blocks of a better tomorrow. By collaborating with each other and harnessing our collective strength and resources, we will be able to create a better and brighter future for our loved ones and for all generations to come. The measure of us as individuals will be based on how effectively we have utilized our time in the world. It will not be based on how long we have lived, but on how well we have lived. Our life span is really an accumulation of minutes and hours, and how effectively we have utilized our allotment of time to achieve meaningful goals. If we have failed to plan in our lifetime, then we have unfortunately planned to fail. Failure to plan is a guarantee for lack of accomplishment.

We must view life as the stages of a day. In any day there is the birth of the sun at dawn, the peak period of the sun at noon and the decline of the sun at sunset signaling the start of the night. Just as there are cycles of light and darkness in every day, so too will there be cycles of happiness and sadness in our lives. Similarly there will be positive and negative experiences on an ongoing basis. We must be armed with the knowledge that our very existence in the world exposes us to cyclic experiences, and we must be prepared to deal with them. Also just as the sun experiences three key periods of dawn, noon and sunset on its journey each day, so too do we experience birth, the journey to peak development and our resplendent glory, and the gradual decline onto the end of our physical existence referred to as death.

As the light of the day fails and we enter the darkness of the night, we are certain that dawn will follow these periods of intense darkness. There is always a birth, a re-awakening, dawn after every night. Our experiences in life will be similar to the daily phenomena of nature highlighting newness. There will always be periods of darkness and negativity, the low tide of our lives. We will be despondent, depressed and full of despair during these occurrences. Just as there is dawn at the end of the darkest night, so too will there be rebirth, re-awakening, freshness and light at the end of the tunnel for all of us.

Our lives will always be cyclic. We will experience ups and downs, happiness and sadness, the thrill of victory and the agony of defeat. Just as night follows day, so too will our personal experiences fluctuate. We must bask in the sunlight during the good times, and prepare ourselves to face the challenges and difficulties during the bad times. With the proper attitude and preparation, we will survive the periods of darkness in our lives. We will rejoice and revel in the positive experiences we create, unlocking the magic of time by becoming masters of our destiny instead of being victims of circumstance.

# 15

## PERSONAL HEALTH AND WELLNESS

There is a general perception that personal health and wellness is something we look at when we get older, well pass the age of forty (40) years. By virtue of youth, many of us are blessed with good health. But with the lack of care, fast-paced lifestyles and pushing ourselves to extreme limits, we wear ourselves down. We must inculcate from an early age a quest to maintain good health and well-being all throughout our lifetime. Our personal lifestyle and habits will lay the foundation for the years to come.

There is a direct impact on the food we eat and on the amount of exercise we get in mapping out our physical well being. Our overall approach to personal care impacts on our fitness levels and health parameters. Our general approach to health in society is reactive in nature. We go to the doctor or personal physician only when something is wrong. We do not have a preventative or proactive approach to our personal health. By the time we do decide to go to the doctor, the damage to our body is very severe. We would have neglected early warning signs from our body, which were telling us that all was not well.

Our attitude to our personal health must be proactive, striving for continuous optimization and improvement and taking note of early warning signs and symptoms. When we carefully review our lifestyles, we pay more attention to our material possessions than to our own bodies. We ensure that we have good stereo and CD systems, DVD players, Computer software, cell phones and impressive automobiles. Our cars are at the center of a lot of attention. We ensure proper oil change, transmission systems, good body job and comfortable interior upholstery. We are meticulous in taking care of our cars but do we pay as much attention to our physical body? Our approach to our cars is very proactive, whereas we are reactive to our personal health. The true vehicle for our movement in the material world is our physical body, a marvel of nature, and unfortunately we do not give it the attention and care that it deserves.

Diet is also critical to our well-being. The choice between the amount of fruits and vegetables in our daily intake, compared to the quota of fast foods and high cholesterol foods directly manifests itself in our physical development. Our source of protein, daily intake of calories and whether we eat meat or not all influence the physical conditions of our body. There are many theories and schools of thought on the types of food we must eat. Some are based on cultural or religious factors, while others are based on scientific research. Ultimately, the choice is ours to review the information and to make an informed decision.

One common factor to the various theories and dietary

proposals is that we must eat in moderation. If we over-indulge and eat excessively, we place additional strain and load on our digestive system. This overwork of our body will eventually lead to the onset of various forms of disease and medical complications.

Illness and disease has been at the centre of medical research for several centuries. Within the last one hundred (100) years, researchers have postulated that over ninety (90) percent of disease is psychosomatic in nature. Mental stress, depression, worry, fear and anxiety are all listed as mental factors which impact negatively on our overall well-being, eventually leading to the onset of different forms of disease.

There is a direct impact of the mind on the physical body. For example, when emotionally we are sad we cry and physical tears flow from our eyes. Intense worry and stress causes ulcers. When we feel fear our muscles tighten and adrenaline flow increases sending the body in a 'fight or flight' mode. Understanding the impact of mental dynamics on the body is the first step towards conquering disease.

We must develop a checklist of factors to monitor our health. The first factor on the list must be the type and amount of food we eat daily. The second must be our body weight to height ratio. Our personal doctors can advise us on the optimum weight for our measured height. The third factor must be an annual certificate of fitness from our doctor. We must perform a medical at least once a year to trend our health and well-being. Our overall health rating leads to the next factor, which is a daily exercise routine. We must consult a physician before we commence any exercise program to guide us on how strenuous to develop our program.

Exercise is a critical factor in establishing good health and fitness. Do we exercise at all? Is our schedule to busy that we do not have the time? Do we feel that we are young and naturally endowed with health so there is no need to exercise? These are common misconceptions and mistakes that pave the way for future medical complications, illness and poor health. Exercise is essential as it improves our circulation, strengthens the muscles, improves our breathing pattern and allows for improved oxygenation of the blood. We must develop a good exercise routine with a few hours of exercise weekly for improved health. We can consult with our doctor, a gym or personal trainer to help tailor a weekly program based on our personal requirements.

Improving our circulation and breathing are critical factors to improving health. Poor blood flow causes lack of proper nourishment of key areas of the body. Poor diet leads to fatty deposits and buildup in our blood vessels that eventually lead to significant restrictions and blockages. Poor breathing means under utilization of the abundant supply of oxygen available for our sustenance. The heart is a continuous pump working non-stop from birth to death. Proper exercise and online maintenance is required for this critical organ. In many chemical industries, there is a spare pump for major processes to act as a backup and to allow for maintenance of the main pump without interruption of the main process. One pump is online with the other on standby. We are not that fortunate with our heart. This loyal organ, a single pump, works continuously for our welfare and well-being. We must do our utmost to take care of it and extend its useful service and life.

We must all do some research into our family medical history. Is there a trend of diabetes, high blood pressure, kidney stones, heart disease or any other illnesses within our family? If so, we need to take extra precaution as there is the likelihood that we may develop these diseases. Our family history is a critical guide and measure on our potential to develop disease. This is the reason that when we apply for insurance and fill out medical forms, no matter how young we are, they always ask questions about the medical condition and history of our mother, father, brothers and sisters are asked.

Some medical conditions are hereditary. Diabetes for example can be passed on from generation to generation. With modern health technology however, diabetes can be controlled and diabetics can lead very normal lives via good diet and lifestyle. There are increased number of products and services available for patients with diabetes. In fact, for conditions such as heart disease, kidney problems and other ailments, there are significantly improved systems and products for the present generation compared to what was available to our forefathers. People are benefiting from these products daily and are leading improved lifestyles.

Stress is a major factor that disrupts health and wellness. Are we worn out, tired, depressed and unhappy? Do we feel mentally drained and yearn for more out of life? Do we struggle to go to work every day, feeling pain and headaches at the mere thought and sight of work? If we have answered yes to these few questions, then we are definitely experiencing abnormal levels of stress.

We cannot achieve good mental dynamics with a body that is physically weak. We must first take steps to re-energize and nourish the body on our path to reduce stress. Once some level of physical nourishment is achieved, we must then work on improving our physical fitness. Walking and light exercise are beneficial in improving circulation throughout the body and establishing improved breathing patterns. Greater oxygenation of the blood reduces toxins in the blood stream and allows us to feel re-energized and re-vitalized.

Proper breathing is the next step as we focus on reducing stress and improving health.

When we are tense, our breathing is fast and shallow. Deep, slow breathing induces a sense of calm and control. Good breathing is an art which is acquired over time, and we must learn to breathe properly. Only then can we achieve maximum benefits of the oxygen so readily available for us in air. The air around us consists of approximately 79 % Nitrogen and 21 % oxygen. Its supply is unlimited and free, and its value is significantly underestimated. If we had to pay for air, we would place more value on its availability. Oxygen is vital in re-energizing our bloodstream and nourishing our brain and physical organs, and an optimum supply is essential. Gases like carbon monoxide form toxins in our system eventually poisoning our bloodstream. A good supply of oxygen is the key to vitality, good health and well-being.

In ancient eastern societies, the art of yoga was taught as a form of harmonizing the physical, mental and spiritual dimensions via control of the senses and proper breathing. Yoga teaches various techniques and methods to strengthen the physical body and improve overall fitness. Within the last century, western society has benefited from this ancient technique of achieving inner peace, relaxation and self-realization. It is one of the most potent forms of eliminating stress, improving mental alertness and wellbeing.

One of the key teachings of yoga is that the physical body is surrounded by an energy field known as its aura. The vibratory energy of an individual's energy field is based on their level of physical, mental and spiritual development. In the metaphysical realm, yoga teaches that there are seven key energy points or centres, each of which is known as a chakra. The chakra is analogous to a wheel that revolves around a centre and unfolds individual vortices. When many rivers meet, a whirling vortex of force is created. The chakra is therefore best described as an energy centre where life forces meet. In ancient literature, there are seven chakras in the human body. The first chakra is located at the base of the spine, the second at the reproductive organs, the third at the solar plexus, the fourth at the heart, the fifth at the throat, the sixth at the eyebrow and the seventh at the crown of the head. The particular site of each chakra corresponds to the body's major biological systems. Based on this relationship, the first chakra is linked to excretion, the second to reproduction, the third to digestion, the fourth to circulation, the fifth to respiration and the sixth and seventh to the functions of cognition and mental dynamics.

The study of the chakras and language on the subject is highly metaphysical. There are several analogies to the physical realm relating to unfolding the energy of the human body. The chakras are symbolic of energy centres or the wheels of life which maintain harmony, balance and well-being at the physical, mental and spiritual level. Further study of the subject will reap tremendous understanding of the major biological systems of the body, and on achieving techniques to improve fitness and health.

The fast pace of modern living induces greater levels of stress and anxiety in modern society. The majority of society faces the morning rush hour via taxis, buses, trains, subways, high speed rail, traffic and congestion. Personal stress levels soar during these periods. A hectic day at school or work is followed by another rush to get back home. We are constantly in a hurry, rushing back and forth to go somewhere, to do something. This is causing havoc within our bodies. We have to regain control of our lives and take positive measures to control our daily stress.

Two of the major factors impacting on the health of youth are alcohol and cigarettes. Over fifty percent of youth in society consume alcohol, smoke cigarettes or do both. As mentioned earlier, the majority of people are gifted with good health at youth. Unfortunately, this is eroded by lifestyles that include alcohol and cigarettes. Alcohol destroys the brain cells, damages the kidney, liver and other internal organs and causes loss of control of motor skills and senses when an individual becomes intoxicated. Medical research has identified the clear link between cigarettes and lung cancer. Amidst all the statistics, and medical facts available, youth continue to indulge in alcohol and cigarettes at an alarming proportion. These two factors are major causes of physical damage to the precious generation of youth in society.

Drunken driving and the senseless loss of life on roadways is part of the legacy of alcohol. International trends continue to see an alarming increase in the loss of young life caused by driving under the influence of alcohol. Many young people who start drinking socially continue this habit into adulthood with negative consequences on the physical body. Whereas cocaine, marijuana and ecstasy cause major damage to the physical body, the impact of alcohol and cigarettes are significantly underestimated. The fight against hard drugs must continue, but the battle to free youth from the shackles of alcohol and cigarettes must intensify.

HIV / AIDS infection rates continue to be a major challenge in the twenty-first century. International statistics indicate the highest level of cases in Sub-Saharan Africa followed by the Caribbean. Apart from allocating increased funds for research and discovering a cure for the disease, additional strategies are required in the battle against HIV / AIDS. Governments worldwide must increase funding for sex education and reproductive health programs, and more outreach programs are required for rural areas and neglected communities. Awareness programs, healthy lifestyles, more informed choices and self-control are essential in the battle against HIV / AIDS.

Promiscuity and multiple sexual relations continue to cause the exponential growth of HIV / AIDS cases globally. Greater moral education and guidance programs are required to guide youth on managing personal relationships and sexual unfolding. The urge for sexual experiences and encounters are accentuated in youth due to hormonal changes and the need for new personal experiences. Greater programs for peer-counseling and youth support networks are required in helping youth to understand their sexuality, their bodies and how to manage personal relationships. The approach to moral education and greater self-control must be further explored as part of the quest to resolve the challenge of HIV /AIDS.

During youth, we are bubbling with energy and vitality. During our teenage years, we spend a significant amount of time at school acquiring education and laying the foundation for our future. During our early twenty's, we enter the world of work, starting new careers and professional experiences. Some youth start work in their late teenage years, getting an early start to the fast pace and demands of the workplace. As we commence this stage of life, many of us get caught in the vicious cycle of hectic work schedules, ad hoc eating and sleeping patterns, total focus on tight deadlines and work commitments and eventual burnout. We need to take steps to regain control of our lives and ensure that we achieve balanced health and wellness.

As we work towards good health, we must always remember the primary importance of the quantity and types of food we eat. Based on our personal condition and preferences we should liase with a doctor and dietician to develop our optimum diet.

Of all the various diets in society, there are a few key points of universal wisdom. The first is to drink copious amounts of water. The recommended amount is a minimum of eight glasses a day, to keep the body hydrated and to improve the removal of waste from the body. The second point is that moderation is the key. We must eat moderately, and strike a balance between the amount of healthy foods and fast foods we ingest. The third point is to take a tablespoon of honey every day. Honey has a healing effect on our body and is absorbed very easily in our digestive system. The ancient Egyptians revered honey for its healing benefits. The fourth point is to eat fresh fruits and vegetables for vitamins and minerals. The fifth key point is that garlic in our foods is a valuable source of health and vitality. We should consult our personal doctor or dietician for confirmation of all recommendations to out diet.

As stated before, we must minimize our alcohol and cigarette consumption with a long term goal to eliminate usage totally. Alcohol damages the brain, heart, liver, kidneys and almost all of our major organs. Cigarettes and smoking accelerate cancer. Let us not wait until we are aged fifty and a doctor orders us to stop taking these substances, and stop usage now. Apart from the physical benefit to our bodies, financially we can recover valuable income via reduced expenditure for these substances.

We need to allocate time for rest and relaxation. Many of us have forgotten the art of relaxation. We need to spend more time doing the things that we enjoy. We should get closer to nature by visiting a nature resort, going to a beach, a lake or a fishing pond. A bath in the ocean has miraculous regenerative effects upon the body. The feel of sea breeze blowing softly on our face, the gentle sound of the waves undulating, the light salty taste of the air, all have a revitalizing impact on our body. Spending more time with family and loved ones also has a beneficial effect on our well-being. If we enjoy cinema, theatre, the arts, we should take time out to indulge in these pleasures.

Leisurely walking is also an invaluable form of relaxation and stress reduction. Apart from the physical benefits of improved circulation, blood supply and breathing, walking allows us quiet time for contemplation and reflection. It allows us time for quality thinking, introspection and self-analysis, giving us time for ourselves away from the normal demands of daily living. Walking is highly recommended for improving health and wellness.

We must develop the art of breathing. Whether we contact a certified yoga instructor, or acquire literature on the ancient art form of yoga, we must learn to breathe properly to improve health and fitness levels. We must also examine our family history and adopt a preventative approach to health rather than a reactive one. We must schedule annual checkups and blood tests to monitor our cholesterol, sugar level and other key factors.

We must seek to do something beneficial to society and those around us. Nothing is more gratifying than making a meaningful contribution to society, which has a lasting positive impact and benefit to our fellow human beings. Whether we take time out to teach people less fortunate than us, contribute to educational funds for children, we can all find some area wherein we can make a contribution.

We must constantly keep the mind active by reading regularly. Mental fitness is a guaranteed way to improve the quality of our life. Just as the physical body requires exercise to keep fit, the mental body requires regular exercise to keep in shape. We must read diverse literature to keep our minds active and challenged. Learning new skills and stretching ourselves mentally will invigorate us to higher levels of overall fitness and alertness.

One of the key things we have forgotten as a society is the ability to laugh and be happy. The world around us has become so serious that many of us do not have an opportunity to laugh. We need to visit a cinema or theatre with a hilarious comedy and experience a hearty session of laughter. This is one of the best medicines for the spirit. Laughter induces very good states of relaxation and is an excellent remedy for eliminating stress. We must once more smile and learn how to be happy.

These are just a few guidelines on maintaining physical health, fitness and wellness. A holistic approach is required to ensure harmony of body, mind and soul. We must work proactively towards better physical, mental health and well-being. We must develop a solutions-oriented attitude and approach to life. By adopting a preventative philosophy and taking care of our physical bodies from the stage of youth, we can improve the quality of our life as we get older, and significantly reduce disease and illness. By improving our health, and extending our lives, we will be able to make a more meaningful contribution and lasting impact on society for the benefit of generations to come.

# EMPOWERING THE SPIRIT

# 16

# THE CHALLENGE OF CHANGE

The only constant in life is change. Personally, professionally, mentally and spiritually, we are constantly challenged by change and have to adapt to new conditions or situations. Every second of our lives we experience change. Our body is constantly evolving and transforming. At every moment new cells are being formed, blood is circulating throughout our body, transporting food and oxygen, and various physiological and biochemical changes are taking place within us. Our Digestive, Circulatory, Nervous and Respiratory systems undergo a symphony of change continuously.

We must embrace change as the very essence of life. New thoughts, ideas and impressions flow through our mind as we experience a continuous current of mental activity. Our mind is in continuous flux adapting to the changes around us. Life is very dynamic. Stagnation is symbolic of death and decay. If we remain the same, and are resistant to change, we become stunted and inhibited in our total development.

Each day brings forward new challenges and obstacles. If we lack flexibility, we will become very stressed and depressed, as we will be unable to cope with new challenges. Life is not about what happens to us, but how we deal with what happens to us. We need to develop courage to face all of our fears and to successfully overcome them.

As students for example, every year we move to a higher form / grade involving new work of greater complexity and difficulty. We move from Kindergarten to Primary, Secondary and eventually Tertiary education. Some of us will enter University, Trade school or higher institutions of learning. This is an essential element of the cycle of change, the continuous progression or movement from one level to another.

In the world of work, we are challenged by a rigorous cycle of change. Organizational transformation, restructuring, rightsizing and downsizing are all components of this cycle of change. These create new stress levels and challenges for the work force. New work procedures, management styles and organizational systems are other key components which employees must develop the flexibility to handle. Voluntary Separation (VSEP), Voluntary Termination of Employment (VTEP) and retrenchment are also part of the phenomena of organizational change presenting new challenges to personnel.

We must manage change, or we will be managed by change. If we are unable to cope with the changes in our immediate environment, we start to lose control of our lives. When this occurs, we become disoriented, depressed and unhappy with our personal situation. We must embrace change as an opportunity for growth, advancement and progress. We must develop a positive attitude and perspective towards change, and regain control of our lives.

When we look at a giant tree in a garden, there are many lessons we can learn by analyzing the different stages of development. The giant tree was once a little seed that was planted in the depths of the ground. It initially struggled in the dark for nutrients to sustain growth. Through fertile soil, water and sunlight, it evolved into a plant and then a small tree. With time, it weathered the elements of intense rain, heat, cold, wind and other external challenges and continued its growth upward to the heavens. With roots planted firmly in the ground, it spread its branches high overcoming all limitations on its journey to become a giant tree.

Change was an essential component in the life of this tree. Change is an essential component of our personal evolution, and is critical for us to move from a lower level of life to a higher plane of existence. Resilience to the different challenges presented by change is just as important. Just as the tree was once a seed struggling in the depths of the earth, so too we are sometimes at a low point in our lives before we commence the progression towards prosperity and success. We sometimes have to go down before we can go up.

In the petrochemical sector, natural gas on its own is relatively cheap. Through the application of intense heat and pressure, natural gas is converted into intermediate products that are further converted to high value products such as methanol, ammonia and urea. The application of intense heat and pressure is critical to producing these high value commodities. In life, we too must undergo the challenge of intense heat and pressure to emerge as products of high value. It is through intense pressure in the earth that coal is transformed into diamond. We emerge as diamonds in society when we survive the intense pressures of life.

As we get older, the people that we love and are fond of

may no longer be with us. When we leave school, friends may drift apart as we move on to new challenges and career paths. Family and friends may migrate to foreign countries in their quest for higher standards of living. Divorce may cause us to be separated from either one of our parents. The ideal homes that we knew become shattered as our parents may go their separate ways, leaving us trying to understand what happened and how to deal with the trauma.

Sickness, ill health and disease may force those we know to cut back on outdoor activity. The ultimate experience for all of us is the death of a loved one. Whether it is a parent, brother, sister, grandparent, uncle, aunt, husband, wife, child, cousin or friend, death brings a sense of finality and is a permanent change, requiring all of our emotional and mental energy to recover. Professional counseling & guidance, and friends to talk to are important support mechanisms to deal with the death of friends and loved ones.

On the other end of the spectrum is the process of birth. Every newborn child is a positive ray of hope in our fast-paced society. Words cannot truly express the miracle of birth, the profound joy and fulfillment of young, new parents. Many of us have grown accustomed to being children ourselves, with our parents looking after us. When we become parents, it indeed is a life changing event. Our entire outlook on the world becomes different. Our decisions, direction and choices in life no longer impact on us only, but impact upon our children. We must manage our lives to ensure the best for our children and loved ones.

The first three years in the life of a child are the formative years. The innocent curiosity of a young child as it explores and strives to understand the world is fascinating. Through the eyes of a child life is an adventure, with fresh and exciting experiences. We must learn from the attitude of the child and look at the world as full of opportunities for discovery and new experiences. We will be able to rekindle the joy and vitality of daily existence. We must work to foster healthy relationships and share positive experiences with the young child, as these leave permanent and lasting impressions, mentally, emotionally, and psychologically.

We must manage change or we will become overwhelmed by the power of change. Life is a continuous cycle of change and we must develop the art of managing this change. We move from the stages of childhood to youth and then adulthood. Each period brings with it new experiences, challenges and opportunities for our progression. As technology continues to drive the pace of existence, we will be exposed to new systems, programs and inventions that will change our very way of living.

Listening to music evolved from live sessions to cassettes, records, CD's and DVD's. Medical research continues to unlock new techniques to improve health, fitness and wellbeing. We are going to live longer, so we will be exposed to more change over our personal life cycle. Automobiles, telecommunications, genetics, entertainment, art, culture, education systems, software and all conveniences of modern society will undergo rapid change and transformation. Business, trade and commerce will all be impacted upon by Internet technology, and we will move to a paperless society. We must be prepared for the rapid change of the twenty-first century and be ready to embrace the new challenges.

The physical landscape of the earth has undergone continuous change for centuries via erosion and other forms of transformation. In our personal lives, our experiences, encounters and personal events transform our mental and emotional landscape leaving an indelible imprint on our internal environment. The people we meet, our daily encounters all impact upon us positively or negatively. For those who are quiet, shy, and lack self- esteem, society applies brute force upon them, causing them personal turmoil. There will always be those who are more aggressive and harsh, who apply extra pressure on less assertive individuals.

As youth in society, we must always remember that it is our right to life, liberty and happiness. We are empowered to manifest change and impact upon our immediate surroundings and environment. We deserve self-respect, and to be treated with dignity and decorum. No one has the right to insult or abuse us. If we make mistakes, we must accept accountability for our shortcomings. But this does not give anyone the right to treat us as inferior or deficient. We must assert our space in society and confidently exercise our right to contribute to the positive advancement and progress of our fellow human beings.

We must harness change towards our benefit and advantage. In society, there will always be scientific change. This impacts on our understanding of the earth and the universe, and improves our standard of living. We must keep up to date with new systems. There will always be political change. New governments will come to power, new leaders will emerge and new policies will evolve. We must understand the dynamics of national and international politics at any given snapshot in time, as they impact directly on our daily living.

The human being is a constantly evolving creature with many moods, habits and customs. This translates into various social trends and fluctuations that affect our personal interaction and understanding of society. We must be aware of all the social changes. Mentally, we are continuously under-going change. Our personal experiences and subliminal in-fluences affect our moods and feelings. Our mental dynamics allow us to gradually gain greater wisdom and understand-ing, as ultimately, experience is the best teacher.

Fashion will continuously undergo the process of change. We need to feel, look and be different. By nature, we cannot stay the same and will try new styles in personal appearance as the latest fashion trends dictate.

Art, architecture, literature and music will also change to reflect the mood of the times. Art imitates life, and the art-ist will continue to reflect the mood of society via painting, sculpture, poetry, song, drama and dance. Music is the balm that soothes the heart of a restless society, and we will contin-ue to seek solace in the lyrics and melodies of our musicians.

Food, cuisine and culinary patterns will undergo change as our dieticians and chefs strive to improve our health and well being. Studies will guide us on the optimum diet and lifestyle. Many of us through personal introspection or life changing events will transform our dietary habits to prolong life and enjoy better health. As we get older, many of us will stop drinking alcohol, give up cigarettes, cut back on our meat intake, use less salt and adapt to other dietary changes for improved personal health and fitness. Change will be-come a way of life.

As we get older, there will be a greater search to under-stand the meaning of life. We will develop a more philosoph-ic overtone, and search for spirituality as the materialism around us starts to lose its appeal, and we yearn for a higher purpose for existence. We will study ideologies, religions and different philosophies, all in a quest to understand our true meaning and purpose in life.

We must be prepared for change, and when it comes we must embrace it. We must eliminate the fear of change, and harness our energy to positively manage change for our benefit and for the benefit of society. Change is a sign of advancement and growth.

The changes in our lives, positive or negative, are necessary stages on our overall path to advancement and personal evolution. We must derive the benefits and lessons of change and utilize it for elevation to a higher plane of existence. The twenty first century will be an exciting era of revolutionary change, transformation and development of new concepts, ideas and initiatives. We must be prepared for the cycle of change before us, and effectively manage our lives to achieve maximum results.

# 17

## UNLEASING THE SPIRIT

What is the legacy we want to leave for future generations? What footprints would we like to leave on the sands of time? When we pass away, how would we like to be remembered, and what contribution would we have made to society? As we get older, these are some of the thoughts and reflections which go through our mind.

In life, we are generally caught up with the hectic pace of daily existence. We sometimes feel like we are always on the hustle, trying to keep up with multiple challenges. Many times we put off the things we really want to do in life, until we get older. Is this the best approach? We should seize the opportunities before us.

Many of us think that we can do the things we really want when we get older. How are we guaranteed that we will live to a comfortable old age and enjoy the finer things in life? If we do make it to these milestones, will we have the health to do that which we desire? Many of us are gifted with youth, health and strength. We must take full advantage of this wonderful opportunity to go after the finer things in life that we desire. We must use this gift of youth to commence the creation of our legacy.

We all have a higher purpose and meaning in life. We are special individuals who have a contribution to make in the higher scheme of human existence. Many of us do not realize this, and cannot see pass our daily life. We are infinitely greater and better than we think we are. At times, however, we are our worst enemies. We are our worst critics. We have low self-esteem and self-confidence, and cannot see ourselves achieving real greatness and success in life. We think that success is reserved for others, and this lowers our personal drive and level of accomplishment.

We all truly have the power to achieve anything we desire. We deserve to be happy. What really is the true purpose of existence? Is it to accumulate wealth? Is it to achieve good health? At the end of the day, the real purpose of life is for us to be happy. We are all searching for happiness; personally, professionally and financially.

We all yearn for happiness. We want our loved ones to be happy. At a higher, more idealistic level, we want society and those around us to achieve happiness. There is nothing wrong with these hopes. Happiness, success and prosperity are our birthright, and belong to every one of us.

Unfortunately, we are sometimes taught that success and happiness only come after a very long time, after very hard work, struggle, suffering and sacrifice. While this may be one of the paths to success, why can't we achieve this similar goal in a shorter, more enjoyable time frame? What is preventing us from achieving our dreams? The only limit to our advancement, progress and success is the limit we place upon our ourselves. We inhibit our own progress by our thoughts, beliefs and practices.

If we only think of ourselves as struggling and surviving, then we will become caught in this loop of existence. The human mind and the thoughts generated within are magnetic in nature. We attract what we constantly think about. If we generally are negative and pessimistic, we attract negative circumstances and situations. If we are positive and optimistic, we are on the pathway to success. We should not view difficult situations as problems, but only as challenges and opportunities for our development. We will be able to derive meaning for each situation, learn key lessons, and constantly be on a trend of progression.

With a positive attitude and outlook, success will definitely be ours. The question arises, however, as to what do we do when it comes? Many people perceive success as the accumulation of significant wealth and assets. This is only one level of measuring success. Many people who have achieved significant wealth and resources still find themselves wanting more out of life. Even though we may have wealth and can experience all that life has to offer, we still find ourselves yearning for more.

We reach a point where the material comforts and luxuries cannot really soothe our soul, or ease our mind. We are like restless souls in search of comfort and care. It is at this instant that we realize that we are infinitely greater than the physical body which protects us. We are an intricate balance of the physical, mental and spiritual dimensions.

Material wealth caters for our physical comfort, but it is unable to truly take us to the higher realms of mental and spiritual success. It is at times like these, when we are no longer satisfied by the physical comforts and luxuries, that we need privacy and personal space for introspection and reflection. We realize that there is more to life than the accumulation of wealth. Our higher nature calls out to us for inner peace and fulfillment via emotional, mental and spiritual upliftment.

Life is full of important choices. The choices we make will lead us to various paths, and will determine whether we find happiness or not. The power of choice dictates the pace of our personal development and enhancement. Our choices must always be guided by considering the impact of our actions. We must always assess the implications of our different choices and use this as a guide to our final decision.

One of the keys to happiness is to visualize good dreams, and to go out in the world and pursue them. We must never limit ourselves to settling for less. We deserve prosperity, wealth and all round happiness. We must never put off the opportunities of youth until when we get older. Life must be an enjoyable adventure. Each day must be exciting and refreshing, as we venture forth towards our personal hopes and dreams. We must think big and take action to achieve our desires.

Life is full of many challenges and trials. Sometimes we become depressed and disoriented when faced with these difficulties. Challenges are a critical aspect of life, necessary for our personal evolution and growth. We all have the power to overcome these challenges, and we must believe in our ability to do so.

Nature reflects some amazing similarities to our personal lives. The four seasons of the year possess their own unique qualities. Spring is a period of rebirth and rejuvenation. Summer is full of sunshine, gaiety and activity. Autumn is somber, and signals change and gradual decay. Winter is cold, challenging, but also a time for rest and reflection. In our personal lives, there are periods of rebirth and rejuvenation. There are high points when we are very happy and overwhelmed. There are times when we must undergo significant change and transformation. There are points when we feel isolated, lonely and depressed.

Our lives are cyclic, with fluctuations, high points, low points, and continuous change. We must recognize this cyclic nature. We must understand that the different points and seasons of our lives happen for a particular reason, essential for our own development. In searching for meaning to the daily occurrences in our lives, many turn to spiritual teachings and writings for guidance.

People have different concepts and perceptions in the fields of philosophy and religion. In the realm of various religious denominations, religion has become very rigid and ritualistic. Leaders and clerics dictate from the pulpit who has access to God, and who does not. This, unfortunately, has made religious and spiritual teachings available only to those whom the leaders perceive as worthy of this guidance.

With all the philosophy and teachings, we must never forget that life is about action and intention. Every one of us is special in our own way, and we have our part to play in society. We all have a contribution to make in the world. Our actions have a direct impact on society and those around us. Religion teaches that a higher, supreme force created the world with tremendous resources at our disposal. In our own way, with our special talents and gifts, we must use these resources to improve the conditions of society.

It is taught that one of the highest forms of worship to the Supreme Intelligence of the universe is work. Work is worship. Whether we become involved in trade, business, professional or non- professional work, we transform the condition of society by our labour. We must utilize the raw materials of the earth to improve the conditions of society.

Will the world be a better place because we have lived? At the end of the day, this is the critical question that will be used to assess the impact of our lives on society. We must model and shape our lives so that the answer to this question will be a resounding yes. Our goal should be to improve the condition of the world because we have lived. We should walk a path in search of personal liberation and elevation. Rapture and spiritual elevation is not exclusively reserved for one group of people. It is the birthright of very one of us.

In the religion of Islam, there is a saying of the Holy Prophet Muhammad (upon whom be peace) to "Seek Knowledge even in China." For the ancient Arab, journey from Saudi Arabia to China required a significant period of travel. The lesson from this ancient saying is that sometimes we must travel great distances in search of knowledge, and we must be prepared to do so. By travelling the earth to various destinations, we can achieve greater knowledge, wisdom and personal insight.

In ancient times, many philosophers studied an esoteric art known as alchemy in search of one of its highest secrets known as the Philosopher's stone. The Philosopher's stone was believed to be able to transform lead into gold. There have been different types of individuals that have sought after this knowledge, namely those who were only interested in physically converting lead into gold, and those who were interested in the higher dimensions of this concept.

In nature, gold is a metal that has been formed after a very high level of evolution. Our universe is constantly evolving and transforming. The conversion of lead into gold is symbolic of the process of evolution, the transformation of something that is ordinary into a product of higher worth and value. We are all initially like lead, and must strive to evolve and be converted into products of greater worth like gold. We must focus on means of achieving personal evolution in the physical, mental and spiritual realms.

When we achieve personal elevation, we are better able to help those around us improve themselves. To transform society, we must first transform ourselves. Only then can we uplift the conditions of our family, loved ones, friends and society as a whole.

Life is full of many trials and tribulations on the path to personal development. There will be good times, and there will be hard times. But at the end of the day, we should have lived in such a way that we were able to enjoy the journey of life. We all have individual goals, and we are sometimes so fixated on these goals that we are unable to enjoy the journey and path to accomplishment of these goals. We must take time to enjoy the journey, and not only rush on towards the destination.

In the mental realm, there are certain poisonous factors that inhibit our progression and growth. We must eliminate mental poisons and negative thinking. Key mental poisons and inhibitors that must be eliminated include:

| Doubt | Jealousy | Timidity |
|-------|----------|----------|
| Worry | Hurry | Pessimism |
| | | |
| Fear | Low Self esteem | Hatred |
| Anger | Envy | Depression |

We must be prepared for the challenges of life, full of self confidence and assertiveness. In nature, with time and pressure, coal is converted into diamond. Without the pressure, it will remain coal, but by harnessing the forces of nature it is transformed into diamond. Like coal, if we are able to withstand the pressures of life, we can harness the forces of nature to emerge as diamonds in society.

There are a few critical factors that are essential for us achieving unlimited success and prosperity in life. These include:

| | | |
|---|---|---|
| Belief in ourselves | Creative Visualization | Strategic Goals |
| Determination | Attitude | Smart Work |
| Perseverance | Courage | Good Intention |
| Will Power | Knowledge | Action |

The last factor, ACTION, is at the heart of success. With all our theory, philosophy, ideology and personals goals, inaction will doom us to failure before we even start. We must boldly take action on the path to achieving our dreams.

We are all searching for happiness. This yearning drives us every day. We all have our own perceptions and interpretations of what defines happiness. Whether it is money, power, wealth, political strength, religion, spirituality or love, these are all means for people to find happiness. No one can really tell us what makes us happy. We must discover this for ourselves. But at the end of the day, it is worthy that we use the gift of life to discover happiness and make those around us happy.

We must dream big dreams. We must set high goals, and take action to achieve them. We must blaze a trail across the sands of time, so that many years from now when we are gone, they can never forget our names. We must live life passionately, savouring the moments and opportunities that come our way. We must tackle all challenges head on. We must leave a legacy for future generations, and seek to make the world a better place because we have lived. At the end of the day, the world should be a better place because we have lived.

Roger Bissessar has served as a Regional Youth Forum representative of the Commonwealth Youth Programme (1999-2002), and has been involved in strategic planning and programs in Australia, Anguilla, Great Britain, Guyana, St Lucia, Solomon Islands and Trinidad & Tobago. He continues to provide support to motivational and educational programs within the Commonwealth. He is an Associate Member of the Institute of Chemical Engineers (AMIChemE) and a life member of the Guild of Graduates of the University of the West Indies.

More information on the Commonwealth and its programs and agencies are available at its website:

www.thecommonwealth.org

www.ingramcontent.com/pod-product-compliance
Lightning Source LLC
Chambersburg PA
CBHW020440290526
45785CB00002B/949